Praise for *The Whole Foods Diet*

"*The Whole Foods Diet* makes a compelling and engaging case for the many advantages of wholesome, whole foods, mostly plants, across the expanse of human health promotion, the ethical treatment of animals, and protection of the environment. The message is not just right, but itself wonderfully whole and satisfying, informed by science, sense, and personal experience; and extending beyond the what, to all the reasons why, and ways how to make such a diet your own. Anyone hungry for good, actionable advice about eating better should certainly dig in!"

—**David Katz**, MD, founding director of the Yale-Griffin Prevention Research Center

"*The Whole Foods Diet* nails it. The secret to living to 100 is knowing the right foods to eat, learning how to make them taste good, and designing your life so that whole, plant-based foods are your easy, go-to choices. Here is a book that is both wonderfully engaging and that supremely delivers on the promise of Blue Zones—a formula for a vital, long, and healthy life, free of chronic disease."

—**Dan Buettner**, National Geographic Fellow and *New York Times* bestselling author of *The Blue Zones* and *Blue Zones Solution*

"*The Whole Foods Diet* is a unique and long overdue comparison of all of the popular programs advising you to eat fewer animals and more whole grains, vegetables, and fruits. By cutting through the confusion created by minor differences between diet experts, you will achieve decision-making clarity necessary for you to regain your lost health and appearance. Read this book before you look any further for advice on what to eat."

—**John McDougall**, MD, author of *The Starch Solution*, cofounder of the McDougall Program

"*The Whole Foods Diet* is enormously compelling and clear-headed but not doctrinaire or the least bit scolding. After reading it, I came out of the experience with my mind full of the right kinds of facts and my stomach ready for the right kinds of foods to invigorate and nourish me. Even with my long experience with these issues, I learned so much and feel like I have a new plan of action."

—**Wayne Pacelle**, president and CEO, the Humane Society of the United States

"In this lively and entertaining book, John Mackey and his coauthors show that a plant-based, whole foods diet is best for us, better for the environment, *and* a more ethical way of living. If everyone were to read *The Whole Foods Diet*, and eat as the book recommends, we would be living in a healthier, happier, and more sustainable world."

—**Peter Singer**, AC, bestselling author of *Animal Liberation*

"So many people want to improve their diets and take advantage of the power that healthy foods can bring, but they are unsure where to begin. The place to begin is here! *The Whole Foods Diet* explains how to use foods to improve your health and gives you simple steps that make the transition easy."

—**Neal D. Barnard**, MD, FACC, adjunct associate professor of medicine, George Washington University School of Medicine; president, Physicians Committee, Washington, DC

"As a physician who specializes in weight loss, I can tell you that most of the diseases we treat in Western medicine find their origins in what we eat. It still amazes me that something so simple—what we should put in our mouths—has been made so complex. My patients are completely confused, and industry wants it that way. *The Whole Foods Diet* is the perfect guide to simplifying the age-old question: What should we eat to be healthy? John Mackey, founder and CEO of Whole Foods Market, has been at the forefront of bringing the public healthy, wholesome food. He has teamed up with two expert physicians who specialize in using food as medicine. Their combined knowledge creates real-world explanations that make nutritional science seem obvious rather than confusing. They address and dispose of fad diets, and in the end offer an excellent guide to creating a healthy lifestyle. This is a must-read for physicians and for the public."

—**Garth Davis**, MD, medical director Bariatric Surgery at Memorial Hermann Memorial City; assistant professor of Surgery, University of Texas-Houston; author of *Proteinaholic*

"I love everything about this book! John, Matt, and Alona have laid out a program to success that is simple, engaging, and delicious! Follow this road map to health and give yourself the life you deserve."

—**Rip Esselstyn**, author of *The Engine 2 Diet*

"In *The Whole Foods Diet* the trio of Mackey, Pulde, and Lederman have thoroughly examined the multitude of 21st-century food plans and through their research and analysis, derived the thoughtful and balanced choice which offers the public the opportunity for optimal health."

—**Caldwell B. Esselstyn Jr.**, MD, author of *Prevent and Reverse Heart Disease*

"Today, more people actually think it's easier to file their income tax on their own than it is to choose healthy food. We are that confused about healthy eating. And yet, as this marvelous new book, *The Whole Foods Diet*, makes abundantly clear, there is in fact a compelling consensus among unbiased health professionals about what foods cause illness, and what foods bring wellness. I would not be surprised if *The Whole Foods Diet* becomes the definitive work on how to eat for a long, healthy, disease-free life. It's that clear. And it's that good."

—**John Robbins**, author of *Diet for a New America* and many other best sellers, president of the Food Revolution Network

"What a great book! How can anyone who reads this not recognize the logic, clarity, and consensus of nutritional science that leads to clear and irrefutable guidelines for superior health?"

—**Joel Fuhrman**, MD, six-time *New York Times* bestselling author; president, Nutritional Research Foundation

"*The Whole Foods Diet* captures the spirit of an exciting new movement—a bottom-up revolution of people who are using the wisdom of good science and the power of nutritious food to take back their health, reverse disease, and live a long life. Read this wonderful, informative book and be inspired to join them!"

—**Michael Greger**, MD, bestselling author of *How Not to Die*

"John Mackey is one of the great food visionaries of our time. From the founding of Whole Foods Market thirty-seven years ago to *The Whole Foods Diet* today, he's arguably done more than anyone else in moving America toward a healthier, more humane, plant-based lifestyle. Get ready, because this book just may begin the journey that will change the rest of your life for the better."

—**Kathy Freston**, *New York Times* bestselling author of *The Book of Veganish*, *The Lean*, and *Quantum Wellness*

THE
WHOLE
FOODS
DIET

THE WHOLE FOODS DIET

The Lifesaving Plan for Health and Longevity

John Mackey, Alona Pulde, MD, and Matthew Lederman, MD

Foreword by Dean Ornish, MD

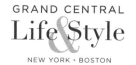

GRAND CENTRAL
Life & Style

NEW YORK • BOSTON

Grand Central Life & Style

Hachette Book Group
1290 Avenue of the Americas, New York, NY 10104

grandcentrallifeandstyle.com

twitter.com/grandcentralpub

First Edition: April 2017

Grand Central Life & Style is an imprint of Grand Central Publishing. The Grand Central Life & Style name and logo are trademarks of Hachette Book Group, Inc.

The publisher is not responsible for websites (or their content) that are not owned by the publisher.

Whole Foods, Whole Foodie, Whole Foods Market, and Eat Real Food are the trademarks of Whole Foods Market IP, L.P.

The Hachette Speakers Bureau provides a wide range of authors for speaking events. To find out more, go to www.hachettespeakersbureau.com or call (866) 376-6591.

Print book interior design by Waterbury Publications Inc., Des Moines, IA
Library of Congress Cataloging-in-Publication Data
Names: Mackey, John, 1954- author. | Pulde, Alona, author. |
Lederman,
Matthew, author.
Title: The whole foods diet : discover your hidden potential for health, beauty, vitality & longevity / John Mackey, Alona Pulde, MD and
Matthew
   Lederman, MD ; foreword by Dean Ornish, MD.
Description: First edition. | Boston : Grand Central Life & Style, 2017.
Identifiers: LCCN 2016054432| ISBN 9781478944911 (hardback) | ISBN 9781478975007 (audio download) | ISBN 9781478944898 (ebook)
Subjects: LCSH: Health--Popular works. | Nutrition--Popular works. | Diet--Popular works. | Medicine, Preventive--Popular works. | BISAC: HEALTH & FITNESS / Healthy Living.
Classification: LCC RA776 .M1153 2017 | DDC 613.2--dc23 LC record available at https://lccn.loc.gov/2016054432

ISBNs: 978-1-4789-4491-1 (hardcover), 978-1-4789-4489-8 (ebook)

Printed in the United States of America

LSC-C

10 9 8 7 6 5 4

To Whole Foodies everywhere

Contents

Foreword

It is a pleasure to write this foreword to *The Whole Foods Diet*. I had long admired John Mackey's visionary leadership of Whole Foods even before we became friends. Now he's teamed up with Drs. Pulde and Lederman to create an engaging, comprehensive guide to healthy eating.

This is the era of lifestyle medicine—that is, changes in diet and lifestyle to treat and even reverse the progression of many of the most common chronic diseases as well as to help prevent them. These changes include:

- a whole foods, plant-based diet (naturally low in fat and refined carbohydrates) like the one described in this book
- stress management techniques (including yoga and meditation)
- moderate exercise (such as walking)
- social support and community (love and intimacy).

In short: eat well, stress less, move more, love more. That's it.

You see it everywhere—after forty years of conducting research in this area, there is a convergence of forces that finally makes this the right idea at the right time:

- Both the limitations of high-tech medicine and the power of lifestyle medicine are becoming increasingly well documented:
  - Data from randomized controlled trials have shown that angioplasties and stents are largely ineffective in most patients who have stable coronary heart disease, whereas my colleagues and I have conducted randomized controlled trials showing that comprehensive lifestyle changes can reverse the progression of even severe coronary heart

disease, without drugs or surgery. There was even more reversal after five years than after one year and 2.5 times fewer cardiac events.

- Data from randomized controlled trials have documented that surgery and radiation do not prolong life after ten years in men with early-stage prostate cancer, whereas my colleagues and I conducted a randomized controlled trial showing that comprehensive lifestyle changes can slow, stop, or even reverse the progression of early-stage prostate cancer, without drugs or surgery. (There is a relatively small subset of men who have especially aggressive forms of prostate cancer who benefit from surgery or radiation, but most men are much more likely to die *with* prostate cancer than *from* prostate cancer.) Also, surgery and radiation can maim men in the most meaningful ways, often causing impotence and incontinence at huge personal and economic costs.

- Our genes are a predisposition, but our genes are not usually our fate. We also found that changing lifestyle actually changes your genes—these lifestyle changes turn off (down-regulate) hundreds of oncogenes that promote prostate cancer, breast cancer, and colon cancer in only three months. In a recent study of men and women at high genetic risk for heart disease, a favorable lifestyle was associated with a nearly 50% lower relative risk of coronary artery disease than was an unfavorable lifestyle. Good lifestyle overcomes bad genes.

- Our latest research found that these diet and lifestyle changes may even lengthen telomeres, the ends of our chromosomes that control aging. We conducted a study with Dr. Elizabeth Blackburn, who was awarded the Nobel Prize in Medicine for her pioneering work with telomeres. As our telomeres get shorter, our lives get shorter and the risk of premature death from a wide variety of diseases increases correspondingly. We found that these comprehensive lifestyle changes lengthened telomeres, thereby beginning to reverse aging at a cellular level.

- Data from randomized controlled trials has shown that lowering blood sugar with drugs does not reduce premature mortality or cardiovascular events, but lowering blood sugar with diet and lifestyle is better than drugs in both preventing and treating type 2 diabetes.

- Because of these findings, Medicare began providing coverage for our lifestyle medicine program for reversing heart disease, and most commercial insurance companies followed suit. Changing reimbursements changes medical practices and even medical education, making it sustainable for physicians to counsel patients on diet and lifestyle changes like the ones described in this book.
- Two years ago, Dr. Kim Williams (president of the American College of Cardiology) learned that his own cholesterol level was very high. Rather than go on a lifetime of cholesterol-lowering drugs, he reviewed the literature to see what alternatives might exist, came across our research, and went on our lifestyle medicine program, including a whole foods, plant-based diet. His LDL cholesterol fell by 50% without drugs. Earlier this year, Dr. Williams convened the ACA's first-ever seminar on lifestyle medicine at their annual scientific sessions. Several hundred cardiologists attended.
- In January 2017, Anne Ornish and I offered the first three-hour workshops on lifestyle medicine at the The World Economic Forum annual meeting in Davos.

Many people tend to think of advances in medicine as high-tech and expensive, such as a new drug, laser, or surgical procedure. We often have a hard time believing that something as simple as comprehensive lifestyle changes can make such a powerful difference in our lives—but they often do.

In our research, we've used high-tech, expensive, state-of-the-art scientific measures to prove the power of these simple, low-tech, and low-cost interventions. These randomized controlled trials and other studies have been published in leading peer-reviewed medical and scientific journals.

The Whole Foods Diet captures this growing movement, bringing together in one book the wealth of evidence for the power of a whole foods, plant-based diet. For example, a new study found that animal protein dramatically increases the risk of premature death independent of fat and carbs. Transcending the ideological debates that rage in the world of diet and nutrition, and cutting through the myths often promoted by special interest groups, fad diets, and the popular media, *The Whole Foods Diet* makes a compelling argument that eating well is not as confusing as it seems.

The book features the commonsense voices of doctors, researchers, scientists, and patients, all attesting to the power of eating a whole foods, plant-based diet, and it offers a wealth of practical guidance to make the transition to a healthier lifestyle.

And what's good for you is good for our planet. What's personally sustainable is globally sustainable.

To the degree we transition toward a whole foods, plant-based diet, it not only makes a difference in our own lives, but also makes a difference in the lives of many others across the globe. That imbues our dietary choices with meaning beyond ourselves. And if it's meaningful, it's sustainable.

Many people are surprised to learn that animal agribusiness generates more global warming due to greenhouse gases than all forms of transportation combined. More than half of US grain and nearly 40% of world grain is fed to livestock rather than consumed directly by humans. In the United States, more than eight billion livestock are maintained, which eat about seven times as much grain as is consumed directly by the entire US population.

It takes about ten times as much energy to eat a meat-based diet as it does a plant-based diet. Producing 1 kg of fresh beef requires about 13 kg of grain and 30 kg of forage. This much grain and forage requires a total of 43,000 liters of water.

So, to the degree we choose to eat a plant-based diet, we free tremendous amounts of resources that can benefit many others as well as ourselves. We have enough food in the world to feed everyone if enough people were to eat lower on the food chain. I find this very inspiring and motivating. When we can act more compassionately, it helps our hearts as well.

And the only side effects are good ones.

Dean Ornish, MD, founder and president, Preventive Medicine Research Institute; clinical professor of medicine, University of California, San Francisco; author, *The Spectrum* and *Dr. Dean Ornish's Program for Reversing Heart Disease;* ornish.com

Introduction

by John Mackey

Breakfast: Cocoa Puffs and milk or bacon and eggs; orange juice from frozen concentrate.

Lunch: Plain hamburger with mustard and mayonnaise, French fries, and a chocolate milkshake or soft drink.

Dinner: Fried chicken, pot roast, or mac and cheese; potatoes; milk; dessert.

My childhood diet wasn't exactly the stuff that nutritional dreams are made of. Neither were my food choices uncommon. Growing up in Houston, Texas, in the 1950s and 1960s, I ate the Standard American Diet of the era, though a particularly narrow version of it. I didn't even eat pizza, which, as I look back today, seems strange. I certainly didn't eat any vegetables (with the exception of potatoes), and honestly, I didn't understand why anyone would. My saving grace may have been that I ate some sweet fruits, such as bananas, apples, oranges, and grapes, which helped give my otherwise deficient diet a much-needed boost of fiber, vitamins, minerals, and antioxidants.

I don't blame my parents—they didn't know any better. That was the era of TV dinners and fast food, when America was unreservedly embracing the conveniences that modern technology made possible, with little awareness of their hidden health costs. Thankfully, public awareness of diet and health has evolved since then, and we have so many more opportunities today to make informed choices about what we feed ourselves and our families. That makes it all the more shocking that a large percentage of Americans still eats a diet that is nutritionally not so different from my childhood menu. For example, 96% of Americans don't reach the USDA's minimum recommended daily intake of 2.5 to 3 cups of vegetables[1] (which in itself is on the low side, in my opinion). The Standard American Diet consists of about 54% highly processed foods, 32% animal products, and just a paltry 14% fruits, vegetables, legumes, and whole grains.[2] When you consider that French fries are counted in that 14%, the picture gets even worse. And it's taking a tremendous toll on our health: 69% of adult Americans are overweight and 36% are obese,[3] and this is leading to an epidemic of chronic disease.

If you've picked up this book, you're likely already aware of these issues. These statistics aren't just numbers to you—they may include yourself or people you know and love. I'll make an educated guess that you're not living on fried chicken and Coke—you're already trying to make health-conscious choices about how you nourish yourself and your family. But you've probably also discovered how challenging it can be to know what the right choices are. Yes, we have much more information today than my mother had when she served up frozen TV dinners, but we don't always know how to make sense of it. In the space of just a few decades, we've gone from information blackout to information overload, with thousands of books and websites and legions of newly minted experts telling us what we should and shouldn't eat.

Despite the sobering statistics, I'm optimistic about the potential for change in individual lives and in our culture at large. As I see every day at Whole Foods Market, consumer consciousness—the most powerful engine of change—is shifting to embrace more sustainable, more ethical, and more organic foods. In my own lifetime, although the health of our nation has arguably gotten worse, our *health potential* has actually increased. With the incredible selection of fresh fruits and vegetables and other healthful whole plant foods available to us year-round, we have the potential to be the healthiest human beings who have ever lived on planet Earth. Plus the nutritional knowledge that is available to most of us today, *if we act on it,* makes it reasonable to aim to live to be one hundred years old, and avoid falling prey to heart disease, cancer, diabetes, and other chronic conditions. My parents' generation couldn't say that. They didn't have access to the knowledge, or the choices, that we have now.

My goal with this book is to empower you—with information, options, and inspiration—to reach your highest health potential. If that doesn't inspire you, you might want to take a moment to ask yourself why. I often hear people say, "I don't want to live to be a hundred!" But what they're really afraid of is getting old and sick. It's not life span but *health* span they're concerned with. When I ask them, "Would you want to live to a hundred if you were healthy, vital, and free of disease?" they say, "Of course!" And I believe this shouldn't be a pipe dream, for most of us. Yes, there are genetic and environmental factors we can't control, and accidents can befall anyone. But we do have more control over our health than ever before, and if we focus on that enormous potential, we just may be able to thrive all the way to the ripe young age of one hundred. The key to unlocking it, as I will explain in this book, is a whole foods, plant-based diet.

My Own Health Journey

How did the kid who never touched a vegetable end up founding America's biggest natural foods supermarket company and writing a book on whole foods, plant-based eating? My relationship to food, like many things in my life, progressed through a series of awakenings. The first came at age twenty-three, when I moved into a vegetarian co-op. This was a radical step for me because, while my food horizons had expanded a little since I had left home, I still had not embraced the idea of eating anything green, and I certainly wasn't vegetarian. However, my growing countercultural interests convinced me I'd meet interesting people in the co-op.

To say I was pleasantly surprised would be an understatement. I discovered that there was a whole wide world of food that was fascinating and delicious. I learned not only to eat but to love vegetables and became the very opposite of my picky childhood self—someone who relished trying new foods and experimenting with the incredible diversity of global cuisine.

I also began to read about natural foods, and soon they became a passion. I had found my life purpose, although I didn't know it at the time. Before long I became the food buyer for our small co-op—my first taste of the food business. Soon after, I took a job at the largest natural foods store in Austin, the Good Food Company. I learned the basics of retail and found it gratifying to sell healthy food to people. One day an idea popped into my head: *I could do this. I could start my own store.* The business that would eventually become Whole Foods Market was born just six months later.

My own menu continued to evolve. I had shifted to eating a primarily plant-based diet, but I had gradually, over a couple of decades, begun to include occasional animal foods and more highly processed foods as well. While I was still healthier than most of my friends and family, my weight was slowly creeping up, and my biometrics, such as cholesterol, blood sugar, and blood pressure, were also getting worse as I aged. That slow health decline was halted in 2003 when I made a key decision: to stop eating animal foods altogether. For me this choice was motivated primarily by ethical concerns (which I'll share in chapter 13), but I noticed pretty quickly that my health began to improve. However, I was still eating quite a lot of highly processed foods such as oils, sugar, and refined flours. After a few years, my health improvements began to plateau.

Then a friend gave me a copy of a book that would trigger an awakening for me: T. Colin Campbell and Thomas Campbell's *The China Study: The Most Comprehensive Study of Nutrition Ever Conducted and the Startling Implications for Diet, Weight Loss, and Long-Term Health.* This book recounts what I consider to be one of the greatest nutritional studies ever done (you'll learn more about it in chapter 3), which came to the revolutionary conclusion that a whole foods, plant-based diet has the capacity to greatly reduce or even eliminate chronic diseases such as heart disease, diabetes, and cancer.

As I shifted my own diet to focus on whole plant foods, I saw dramatic improvement and lost weight steadily. In fact, I now weigh the same as I did at eighteen, and I feel better than I did when I was thirty. My total cholesterol dropped from 199 to 135, my LDL cholesterol from 110 to 70, and my blood pressure declined to 110/75. I would soon discover that there were many other respected doctors and scientists coming to similar conclusions as those of The China Study—pioneers of the whole foods, plant-based eating movement. You'll meet many of these "Whole Foodie Heroes" in the pages of this book.

Indeed, it soon became clear to me, as I read every book and nutritional study I could get my hands on, that there is an overwhelming consensus on the optimum diet for health and longevity among true nutritional scientists. To put it simply, *eat more whole foods and fewer highly processed foods; eat more plants and fewer animal products.* So why isn't this common knowledge? That's a complex question. There are enormously powerful industries invested in keeping Americans eating a diet that leaves them fat and sick. And as individuals, we have become accustomed to the "quick fix" of high-calorie foods, often justifying our habits with unquestioned beliefs and convictions that have little scientific basis. The good news is this: the information you need is out there, and as you start to act on it, your own preferences can and will change. In the pages ahead, I hope to help you see beyond the smoke screen of misinformation and discover for yourself that eating right is not as confusing as it seems.

Why I Wrote This Book

I find it horrifying that so many Americans today are obese, chronically ill, and slowly dying because of the food they eat. We are a nation beset with illnesses that saddle us with expensive and unnecessary healthcare costs. We pour money into medical research, when in reality most of these diseases have already been proven preventable. We falsely imagine that we have no power to protect ourselves from frightening diagnoses like cancer, diabetes, and heart disease. Our medical system has done some truly wonderful things in the last century, but the chronic diseases of today are far more preventable and even reversible than most doctors realize. I was inspired to write this book because I want more people to know how powerful they truly are when it comes to their own health.

I also feel compelled to do what I can to highlight the good news—the growing whole foods, plant-based movement that is emerging in our culture. The world of diets has an unfortunate tendency toward tribalism, and we can sometimes miss the broad agreements by focusing too much on the minor differences. I see this happening too often in the plant-based community. Individual doctors brand their particular protocols and distinguish themselves from each other—this one encouraging eating more starches, that one more vegetables; this one rejecting all oils and high-fat foods, that one allowing some nuts and seeds; this one insisting on 100% plants, that one incorporating a small amount of animal foods. What strikes me, however, when I look at these diets is that they are all promoting the same broad patterns. And when it comes to our health, it's the overall dietary pattern that makes all the difference. Get the big picture right, and there's room for variation on the particulars. By highlighting so many of these different proponents of whole foods, plant-based eating in the book, I hope to shed light on the broad consensus that exists among them, remove unnecessary confusion, and promote unity among the various healthy diet tribes.

Finally, I want to share with you my own conviction that diet change doesn't have to be about deprivation, limitation, and loss of pleasure. On the contrary, I hope this book will open up new horizons in your consideration of what you *can* eat and what that food can do for you. You may choose, for your own reasons, to eat a 100% plant-based diet, but I do not believe you need to make that choice in order to live a long and healthy life. What I do believe—and it's a belief that is backed by the best science available—is that eating 90+% whole plant foods, and avoiding highly processed foods, is the optimal choice for health and longevity. Within those parameters you have tremendous flexibility to create a diet that satisfies your needs, nourishes your body, and delights your senses. I hope this book will awaken you to the possibilities that lie on your plate.

I should make it clear that the recommendations made in this book are based on the views of my coauthors and myself, not Whole Foods Market. I'm tremendously proud of the impact that my company has had, both in increasing cultural awareness of food and in offering millions of Americans more options when it comes to making healthy, sustainable food choices. But I'll be the first to tell you that I wouldn't eat many of the products we sell. People often ask me, "John, how come you sell things in your store that you wouldn't eat?" And I remind them that I'm not a dictator, and I don't get to unilaterally decide what Whole Foods Market should sell or what other people should be able to choose to eat. Like all businesses, Whole Foods needs to sell what its customers want to buy, or they will go shop someplace else. What I can do is play my part in helping people be better informed so they can choose wisely for themselves.

The beauty of our modern culture is that we are blessed with an abundance of choices—what we need are the tools and information to help us navigate them wisely. I wrote this book to help you do just that. Wherever you are—whether at a supermarket, the corner store, or your local farmers market; an airport, a cocktail party, or a shopping mall food court—I want you to have the confidence to pick the best available foods with which to nourish your body.

How to Use This Book

This book is divided into three parts. Part I is designed to educate, demystify, and inform you. I hope you'll be surprised and impressed by the sheer breadth of research that supports the shift to a whole foods, plant-based diet. Knowledge is power when you know how to interpret it and see it in context. In these chapters we'll present a synthesis of the best science, and also help you to understand how to distinguish good science from bad. We'll take a closer look at how diet and lifestyle change have been shown to prevent and reverse two of the most common chronic conditions: heart disease and diabetes. And we'll walk you through the most popular dietary trends of today, including the Mediterranean diet, low-carb diets, and the Paleo diet, and show both their strengths and their potential dangers. We'll analyze their claims so you can have an informed conversation with your Paleo friend from the gym or your concerned mother-in-law who thinks you're not getting enough protein. Hopefully, these chapters will answer your questions—the ones you already have and the ones you haven't thought of yet.

Part II is designed to give you practical support for making the transition to the Whole Foods Diet. We'll talk about everyday food choices and offer some simplifying tools for choosing the most nourishing foods. Our list of the Essential Eight foods will help you become a more skillful eater. We'll share some insights into the inner dimensions of this transition—the psychological challenges of diet change. And we'll look at real-life situations that everyone faces—from grocery shopping to travel to eating out—and share the best tips we've learned. Included in this section are helpful lists for shopping and equipping your kitchen.

Finally, in Part III, we invite you to try the 28-Day Eat Real Food Plan! You'll find a day-by-day sample meal plan and more than forty delicious, nutritious, easy-to-prepare recipes to guide you through four weeks of your new lifestyle.

Introducing My Coauthors

I am happy to be joined in this endeavor by two of the most inspiring people I've met during my journey of health education, Dr. Alona Pulde and Dr. Matthew Lederman. (While this introduction and the concluding chapter are in my voice, the rest of the book is very much a joint effort, drawing on our collective expertise and written in "our" voice.) Back in 2011, I watched one of the best documentaries available on whole foods, plant-based eating, *Forks over Knives*, and I was struck by the two young doctors who worked with the film's narrator, helping him change his own diet and track his progress. Based in Los Angeles, they ran a lifestyle medicine clinic where they helped people make dramatic shifts in their health and happiness through changing what was on their plates. I was happy to see a new generation of medical professionals taking forward the work of so many of my heroes.

I would soon have the opportunity to meet Matt and Alona at a weekend conference run by one of those heroes, Dr. John McDougall, whom you'll meet in chapter 7. We quickly bonded over our shared passion for food and health, and a partnership was born that would give birth to this book—and much more. I invited Matt and Alona to join me in creating a series of programs to help the team members at Whole Foods Market improve their health through better nutrition. This series includes an incentive-based program to encourage better food choices and an annual series of "Health Immersions" to educate and empower thousands of Whole Foods team members. I'm very proud of the work we're doing, and I hope this book will serve to extend our impact beyond our team members to millions more health-conscious and concerned Americans.

In the pages that follow, Matt and Alona bring their combined three decades of real-world medical practice with thousands of people like you, and I add my four decades of intensively studying food and diet and being at the forefront of the natural and organic foods revolution. To all of this, we add the invaluable research and wisdom of our heroes in the field, and our shared passion for helping people heal and thrive with whole foods. We invite you to join us, and tens of thousands of other men and women, in dispelling unnecessary confusion and becoming living proof of our human health potential.

PART I

THE WHOLE TRUTH: WHAT WE KNOW ABOUT DIET AND HEALTH

CHAPTER 1

Are You a Whole Foodie?

Defining the Optimum Diet

"[The] evidence is overwhelming at this point.
You eat more plants, you eat less other stuff, you live longer."

—*Mark Bittman, TED talk*

Food. The term is almost synonymous with life itself. We devote more time to procuring food and eating than we do to any other life-sustaining activity except breathing and sleeping. Food is one of our greatest sources of pleasure, and it is one we share with those we love. We eat as a family, a community, a tribe, nourishing our bodies at the same time that we nourish our relationships. Indeed, dining together releases oxytocin, the "love hormone" that stimulates greater human connectivity. While every species must eat, the human imagination has imbued the simple acts of preparing and consuming food with a whole world of emotion and meaning. Food can express love, gratitude, compassion, creativity, and identity. Historically it has formed a building block of culture—cementing alliances, capturing the unique character of a people, marking significant events. Food is celebration. Food is connection. Food is life.

Yet for millions of people, food is also synonymous with stress, weight gain, neurosis, confusion, and even disease. Americans today have the potential to be the healthiest human beings ever to have walked this earth, but we are quite the opposite. 69% of US adults are overweight and 36% are obese,[1] and these numbers have been steadily rising over the past fifty years.[2] 17% of children are obese, and 19% have a diet-related chronic condition.[3] More than one million Americans die every year from heart disease and cancer, conditions widely referred to in the medical profession as "lifestyle diseases." In other words, they are primarily caused by the way we eat and other controllable factors. A shocking 115 million Americans are diabetic or prediabetic.[4]

A recent survey from the Organization for Economic Cooperation and Development compared America to thirty-three other member countries on multiple health factors, including life expectancy and death rates from various diseases, and America came in close to the bottom on almost every one.[5] And we are exporting our bad dietary habits, with obesity and diet-related disease rates rising around the world as developing countries rush to eat just as we do.[6]

Many of us are trying to do better. According to a 2015 survey,[7] 77% of Americans are actively trying to eat healthier and researchers estimate that more than 50% of the population is "on a diet" at any given time.[8] We are eating fewer calories and drinking fewer sugary sodas, and obesity rates may have finally peaked.[9] The organic food moment has only picked up steam since Whole Foods Market took it national in the 1980s and '90s. Numerous healthy-eating initiatives dot America's food landscape, and things that once seemed fringe are becoming commonplace. At this point, however, the green shoots of good news are still crowded out by the bad. Never has there been such variety and abundance of healthy foods available to us, but never has there been so much seemingly conflicting information about what we should and should not eat. Judging by our national health statistics, it would seem that as a culture we are not doing too well at navigating the all-important question we have the privilege of asking: *What should I choose to eat today?*

Our grandparents, our great-grandparents, and the generations before them never had options the way we do. They probably just ate whatever was most readily available—foods that they could grow or obtain from local producers. In many cultures around the world today, this is still the case.

And too many people still struggle simply to get enough to eat. But those of us who are blessed with an abundance of choices have the enviable but serious problem of needing to learn to eat well.

Eating is something every human being does, but most of us don't do it very skillfully. In fact, *skillful* is not a term we tend to associate with eating, but we should. You wouldn't expect to be able to play a sport or a musical instrument very skillfully without dedicated study and practice. The same applies to eating. Just because you've been doing it all your life doesn't mean you've mastered the art of self-nourishment. You may just be eating the way your parents brought you up to eat, or the way your friends eat, without deeply thinking about whether it will help you to achieve your own health and life goals.

Every person today who wants to live a long and healthy life needs to become a skillful eater, and we need to bring up our children to be the same. A skillful eater is one who has studied the best of what nutritional science can teach us about food and the way it affects our bodies. She knows how to see past the fog of confusion created by the media and the latest diet fads. A skillful eater makes informed decisions every day about what he puts in his mouth. And his tastes have evolved, along with his understanding, so that what he loves to eat and what's good for him to eat are one and the same.

The chapters that follow will teach you to become a more skillful eater, in all these ways and more. If you've picked up this book, you've likely already begun that journey of development. You're already asking yourself some variation on the question: What kind of diet should I choose for optimum health, vitality, beauty, and longevity? Maybe you're a lifelong explorer of wellness. Maybe you're a passionate foodie who loves to eat and also wants to be healthy. Maybe you're frustrated, having tried countless diets but failed to achieve your goals. Maybe you've had a health scare and been told you need to change your lifestyle before it's too late. Maybe you're just tired of all the confusion and yearning for some commonsense answers. Whatever brought you here, we hope these pages can offer you the inspiration, clarity, and confidence to become a more skillful eater.

It's Not as Confusing as It Seems

Which is easier: doing your taxes or figuring out how to eat a healthy diet? In a 2012 study, 52% of people chose the former.[10] If you feel confused about the best diet for health and longevity, you're not alone, and it's not surprising. Nutritional science, and the news stories that disseminate it, can make you feel as if you might as well just give up trying to find a simple answer and eat whatever you feel like. For every study about some particular finding related to diet or health, a contradictory one can be found. As you sip your morning coffee and idly wonder whether it's doing you any good, you can easily drum up an article proclaiming coffee's benefits (antioxidants!), another decrying its ills (caffeine!), a third telling you that to feed your brain you should be drinking your coffee with butter, and a fourth arguing convincingly that bone broth is the new coffee. As you contemplate whether to have bacon, pancakes, or a banana for breakfast, you can find studies and books affirming or challenging each option, some telling you why you should skip breakfast altogether, and others declaring it to be the most important meal of the day. And your friends all claim to have the answers—based on books they've read, diets they've tried, and cutting-edge information they heard from a trainer at the gym. It's little wonder so many people are perplexed by the options on their plates.

It's tragic that our country's health is failing so badly, because eating well is actually not as confusing as it seems. There are hundreds of different *philosophies* of eating, and many people and institutions with a vested interest in promoting one or another of them; but when it comes to actual science, there's a surprisingly robust consensus about what foods make us sick and what foods make us healthy. As Walter Willett, MD, chair of the Department of Nutrition at Harvard School of Public Health, and Patrick J. Skerrett, MA, confirm, there are "enough solid strands of evidence from reliable sources to weave simple but compelling recommendations about diet."[11]

Yes, there will always be controversies and contradictions, especially when we focus on the details, and there is a considerable amount that science simply does not yet understand about the complex interplay between the foods we eat and the intricate systems of our bodies. We as authors have spent decades studying this subject, continue to seek out the latest studies, and consider ourselves lifetime students of nutritional science. But the bottom line is simple. What we *already* know—if acted upon—is enough to extend our lives, revolutionize our health, and dramatically reduce our risk of developing chronic diseases. What do we know? It's this simple:

A whole foods, mostly plant-based diet is the optimum diet for health, vitality, and longevity.

What is a whole foods, plant-based diet? Put simply, it is a diet that prioritizes eating whole or unprocessed plant foods; minimizes meat, fish, dairy products, and eggs; and eliminates highly processed foods.

As you'll see, this is not necessarily a vegetarian or vegan diet. We suggest that you eat a *whole foods, ninety-plus percent (90+%) plant-based diet,* which means keeping animal foods (meat, fish, eggs, and dairy products) to 10% or less of your calories. Most importantly, the Whole Foods Diet is not about deprivation, limitation, and loss of pleasure. This is a dietary approach that is inclusive and can be customized for individual needs and preferences. Do you feel attracted to the Mediterranean diet, the Paleo approach, the gluten-free lifestyle, or the vegan ethos? All of these dietary philosophies can be adapted to fit into a Whole Foods Diet framework. Within the parameters of a whole foods, 90+% plant-based diet there is tremendous flexibility to create meal after meal that satisfies your needs, nourishes your body, and delights your senses.

We're hardly alone in coming to the conclusion that this way of eating is optimal. Hundreds of doctors, clinical trials, and epidemiological studies involving millions of people over several decades have confirmed, over and over again, this simple message about food and health. In fact, when Dr. David Katz, a respected researcher in the field and founding director of the Yale-Griffin Prevention Research Center, was asked to compare the medical evidence for and against each of the major dietary trends in the West today—including Paleo, Mediterranean, low fat, low carb, low glycemic, vegetarian, and vegan—his conclusion was this: "A diet of minimally processed foods close to nature, predominantly plants, is decisively associated with health promotion and disease prevention."[12]

In 2015, together with the nonprofit Oldways, Katz convened twenty-one leading nutritionists of varying persuasions—from plant-based advocates such as Dr. Dean Ornish to the father of the Paleo movement, S. Boyd Eaton—to seek "common ground" on dietary best practices. While the assembled experts didn't take it quite as far as Katz's own review, their recommendations pointed in the same direction: "A healthy dietary pattern is higher in vegetables, fruits, whole grains, low- or nonfat dairy, seafood, legumes, and nuts; moderate in alcohol (among adults); lower in red and processed meats; and low in sugar-sweetened foods and drinks and refined grains."[13]

Despite some inherent differences, the experts were not so far apart after all. Almost no one argues, for example, that we should eat highly processed foods, and just about everyone agrees that fruits and vegetables are vital to human health, and we should consume a great deal more of them. (In America, total per-capita consumption of fruits and vegetables was 1.68 cups per day in 2014, a drop from 1.77 in 2009.[14] This is significantly short of the USDA recommendation of 4.5 cups, and we would consider even that to be on the low side.)

Things get somewhat more complicated when it comes to grains, fats, and the overall health profile of meat and dairy products. We will spend much more time in the chapters that follow exploring the science around these specific food groups. But the simple point is that while some degree of confusion certainly exists, there is also significant consensus and agreement.

Katz is unequivocal on this point: "We are not, absolutely not, emphatically NOT clueless about the basic care and feeding of Homo sapiens," he writes. "The fundamental lifestyle formula, including diet, conducive to the addition of years to our lives, and life to our years, is reliably clear and a product of science, sense, and global consensus. Really. You can be confused about it if you want to be, but I advise against it. You will be procrastinating and missing out—because healthy people have more fun."[15]

The science may still be limited, incomplete, even deficient in a few ways, but it is our contention that, approached with an unbiased mind, it speaks with a clear and consistent voice, telling us that the best diet for health and longevity is a whole foods, plant-based diet. There are many dietary variations on this fundamental theme, but, as Katz emphasizes, "the theme is way past debate."[16]

Our conviction in the power of a whole foods, plant-based diet doesn't just come from reading medical journals. We get to witness the results firsthand as well. Each one of us has experienced the transformation of his or her own health as he or she shifted to this way of eating. And at Whole Foods Market, we've had the privilege of watching thousands of team members discover their own health potential. We offer weeklong "immersion" programs free of charge to those who meet the health criteria. Guided by four of our Whole Foodie Heroes—Joel Fuhrman, MD; John McDougall, MD; Scott Stoll, MD; and Rip Esselstyn (with Michael Klaper, MD)—these events are powerful and life changing for many. Often these men and women started out overweight or obese, diabetic, or suffering from high blood pressure, high cholesterol, heart disease, and other life-threatening conditions. During the immersions, many of them have seen dramatic results in even just one week, and have gone on to lose weight and in some cases have completely reversed their diseases. You'll read some of their "Whole Foodie Stories" in the pages ahead.

Defining the Diet

Let's break down the definition of the Whole Foods Diet a little further. There are two key ideas that create the broad parameters for this approach to skillful eating. First, the difference between whole foods and highly processed foods, and second, the difference between plant foods and animal foods. The Whole Foods Diet advises you to follow two simple guiding principles:

1. Eat whole foods instead of highly processed foods.
2. Eat mostly plant foods (90+% of calories).

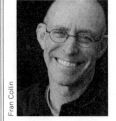

Fran Collin

WHOLE FOODIE HERO
Michael Pollan

"Don't eat anything your great-grandmother wouldn't recognize as food."

Contributions: Pollan's journalistic forays into the world of food, beginning in 2006 with *The Omnivore's Dilemma: A Natural History of Four Meals,* opened millions of eyes to the realities of our industrialized food system and the need to eat real food. His simple rules for eating have become iconic: "Eat food. Mostly plants. Not too much."

Fun facts: Pollan believes in writing from personal experience. This has led him to buy a steer, shoot a boar, and plant a GMO potato in his own garden.

Read this: *In Defense of Food: An Eater's Manifesto*

Learn more: MichaelPollan.com

Follow these two rules and you will essentially follow a dietary pattern that resembles those of some of the world's healthiest and longest-lived populations. Michael Greger, MD, who has done more than anyone we know to aggregate the wealth of scientific evidence for a whole foods, plant-based diet, has summed up its rationale in two simple statements that apply in almost every case: "Plant foods, with their greater protective nutritional factors and fewer disease-promoting ones, are healthier than animal foods, and unprocessed foods are healthier than processed foods."[17]

Food writer Michael Pollan captures the essential point even more succinctly in his three-part manifesto for healthy eating: "Eat food. Mostly plants. Not too much."[18] Although Pollan is a prolific writer who has been instrumental in enlightening millions of people about where their food comes from, these memorable seven words may go down in history as his greatest contribution. He tells us that doctors are now starting to include this phrase in their dietary recommendations to patients—a welcome sign that perhaps a much-needed shift is beginning.

By "Eat food," Pollan means eat whole, real foods instead of processed "food-like substances," as he calls them. "Mostly plants" speaks for itself. Incidentally, if there's one part of his statement we respectfully take issue with, it would be the last: "Not too much." It's certainly true that most Americans consume excess calories and could benefit from moderation. But the beautiful thing about a whole foods, plant-based diet is that if you really follow those first two instructions and eat food, mostly plants, it's hard to eat too much. You'll naturally find yourself satisfied and nourished without overconsuming calories, and you'll experience the joy of no longer having to worry about portion control.

Whole Foods vs. Processed Foods

A whole food means an unprocessed food—a food that is still close to the form in which it grew. It has not been broken down into its component parts and refined into a different form. It's *real* food. As Pollan puts it, "If it came from a plant, eat it; if it was made in a plant, don't."[19]

Sounds pretty simple, right? But if you take this definition to the grocery store, you'll quickly find yourself with a whole new set of questions.

The truth is that, unless you eat it fresh from the garden, almost every food has undergone some form of processing, even if it is only that it has been harvested and its stalks or leaves have been removed. Even whole grain brown rice, a poster child for whole foods, has had its husks removed to make it edible. So if we accept that most food is processed in some way, the question becomes, how much processing is too much? Where do we draw the line on the spectrum between reasonable adaptions that make our food more accessible and adulterations that make it unhealthy?

Journalist Megan Kimble decided to take this question literally when she went a whole year without eating a processed food, while living in New York City. "All foods are processed," she writes in *Unprocessed: My City-Dwelling Year of Reclaiming Real Food*, "but if we understand the difference between an apple and a bag of Chex Mix—and we do—and if the space between the two matters for the health of our bodies and the environment—and it does—then the question of what makes a food too processed also matters."[20]

Kimble took her quest to the extreme—milling her own wheat, extracting salt from the sea, slaughtering a sheep, and milking a goat. We're assuming most readers of this book won't go that far. However, you might start thinking more carefully about what someone else has done to your food and whether it constitutes "too much processing" or not.

Let's say you're looking at a bag of steel-cut oats. They're cut up, so are they a whole food? Common sense tells you they're a lot better for you than the sugary boxed oat cereals down the aisle. But why? In this case there are two reasons. First, while the steel-cut oats may have been cut up, all their parts are still there. None of the important nutrients have been removed in the process. Second, nothing has been added to them—no sugar, salt, oil, or preservatives. So while those steel-cut oats are not *technically* whole, they are so minimally processed that they can be considered a whole food.

Next, let's look at the difference between an olive and a bottle of olive oil. To get from the fruit to the bottle of oil, the olives are ground into a paste, pressed to separate the liquid from the fiber, placed in a centrifuge to drain out water, and then filtered to remove any remaining particles. All of these steps make olive oil a processed food, packed with calories and stripped of nutrients. (If you've been led to believe that olive oil is a health food, you've been misled, as we'll explain in chapter 4.) If you want nutritional benefit, eat the whole olive, with its additional fiber and other nutrients. By the same principle, eating an apple can be wonderfully nutritious; drinking apple juice is much less so. Eating a freshly grilled ear of corn is a perfectly healthy choice, while eating a salted, fried corn chip—well, not so much.

A good definition of a whole food, then, might be a food that retains all its original edible parts, and has not been altered by the addition of other processed ingredients. Once again, Greger offers a succinct summation: "I like to think of 'unprocessed' as *nothing bad added, nothing good taken away.*"[21]

This is by far the best definition we've come across, so with thanks to Greger, we will adopt it for the course of this book. By this measure you can

Whole Foods vs. Processed Foods

While these do not apply in every case, here are some general rules you can use to help distinguish between whole and processed foods:

Whole Foods:

- are close to their original state
- spoil faster
- are things your great-grandparents would have recognized as food
- don't usually have ingredient lists, or, if they do, have short ones
- are often sold without packaging
- are often found around the perimeter of the grocery store

Highly Processed Foods:

- bear little resemblance to their original state
- do not spoil easily
- are things your great-grandparents probably wouldn't recognize
- have (often long) ingredient lists
- are packaged or boxed
- are often found in the center of the grocery store

throw your bag of steel-cut oats or rolled oats in the cart with no further thought, but we hope you will pass by the sugary oatmeal cookies without a second glance.

When it's not possible to eat foods in their completely unprocessed form, make sure the processing is minimal. For example, take the difference between whole wheat pasta, made from whole grains, and white pasta, made from refined white flour with most of its fiber removed. Or the difference between peanut butter, with no added oils, sugars, or salt, and the kind of peanut butter that most American kids grow up on, packed with added sugar, salt, and fat, and with much of its fiber removed. In each example, both are processed, but there's a world of difference between them. Real foods, eaten close to their whole and natural state, are optimally beneficial for the body.

To be clear, cooking is a form of processing, but it's also a minimal one. We're not advocating a raw-foods diet. Cooking is a wonderful human invention that often enhances the benefits of foods, makes them easier to digest, and in some cases releases more nutrients. As a general rule, the foods we choose to eat, whether raw or cooked, should be as close as possible to the way they came off the tree, vine, or root.

Plant Foods vs. Animal Foods

Plant foods grow in the ground or on trees or vines—fruits, vegetables, beans and other legumes, grains, nuts, and seeds. They make up much of what we consider *real* food—apples, tomatoes, potatoes, corn, rice, almonds, beans, strawberries, lettuce, and so on. For the Whole Foods Diet, we recommend that 90% or more of your calories come from plant-based food. Once again, this is not a vegan diet (unless you choose to eat 100% plants for personal reasons), but it is a diet that includes far fewer animal foods than the Standard American Diet.

Animal foods come from the flesh or organs of animals (including mammals, birds, fish, and insects) or are produced by the animal, such as milk products and eggs. For the Whole Foods Diet, we suggest that 10% or less of your daily calories come from this category of foods. As a general rule, that means that meat, fish, dairy products, eggs, and other animal foods are eaten occasionally, as side dishes or condiments—not as the primary calorie source in every meal. You might add some goat cheese to your salad, eat the occasional omelet for breakfast, add shrimp to your stir-fry, or even treat yourself to a small grass-fed steak to celebrate a special occasion, but your daily staples should be whole plant foods. In some respects, this harkens back to more traditional diets, in which it was common to eat animal foods sparingly or occasionally, on particular feast days, not as the centerpiece of every meal. The Whole Foods Diet revives this healthy tradition.

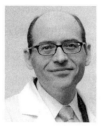

WHOLE FOODIE HERO
Michael Greger, MD

"We should all be eating fruits and vegetables as if our lives depended on it—because they do."

Contributions: Dr. Greger claims to read every issue of every English-language nutrition journal in the world "so busy folks like you don't have to." What's more, he distills the information into easy-to-understand daily blogs and videos on his website NutritionFacts.org, a paragon of trustworthy information about health and diet.

Fun facts: Dr. Greger's grandmother was a patient at the Pritikin Longevity Center in the late 1970s. After multiple heart surgeries, she'd been declared beyond medical help at age sixty-five, but after switching to a plant-based diet, she lived another thirty-one years, inspiring her grandson's passion for food as medicine.

Read this: *How Not to Die: Discover the Foods Scientifically Proven to Prevent and Reverse Disease*

Learn more: NutritionFacts.org

The best research on health, disease, and longevity clearly shows that people who eat a diet of *predominantly* plant foods have dramatically better long-term health outcomes than those who eat a diet heavy in animal foods. Some doctors and nutritionists, including some of the people we feature in this book, will argue that this means we should eat 100% plant-based diets. We as authors have all made that choice, but we want to be clear that we've made it for personal reasons (which we'll return to in chapter 13). We remain open-minded as to what future research will uncover about the potential benefits and risks of including limited amounts of animal products in a healthy diet (see page 150 for further discussion). For now, based on our best reading of the accumulated science, our recommendation is that a whole foods, 90+% plant-based diet is optimal for health and longevity.

We'll return to this topic throughout the chapters ahead and share some of the research and arguments that have led to our recommendations. As you'll see, observations of the world's longest-lived populations, along with various other compelling studies, make a persuasive argument for significantly reducing one's animal food intake, particularly when coupled with the growing evidence for the link between high levels of animal foods and chronic disease. Plant-based diets have been shown to prevent and reverse many of the chronic conditions that afflict millions of Americans, including diabetes and heart disease. Eating more whole plants, in all their wonderful and varied forms, is an undeniable route to health and longevity.

A Whole Food Is More than the Sum of Its Parts

Protein. Fat. Carbohydrates. If you're someone who pays attention to your dietary choices, these are probably terms you use or think about daily. And they are likely associated with certain value judgments. Protein is good! Carbohydrates are bad! Fat is . . . well, we used to think it was bad, but these days lots of people are telling us it's good! When Americans think about nutrition, we tend to think in terms of nutrients, not foods. Along with the three macronutrients just mentioned, there are a host of other substances— fiber, various vitamins and minerals, and phytochemicals—otherwise known as micronutrients. Our foods are judged, and marketed, on the basis of their particular combinations of these substances. That's why most of us grew up being told to drink milk for calcium or eat spinach for iron. Pollan calls this perspective "nutritionism," and much of his 2008 book *In Defense of Food* is dedicated to shedding light on this troublesome ideology and its effects.

As Pollan and many others have pointed out, scientists are trained to be "reductionist"—to break things down into variables they can isolate and study. And while this method has contributed in many important ways to the sum of human knowledge, it has a tendency to obscure even as it reveals. Pioneering nutrition researcher T. Colin Campbell sums this up when he writes, "Few scientists are trained to look at the 'big picture,' and instead specialize in scrutinizing single drops of data instead of comprehending meaningful rivers of wisdom."[22]

The overemphasis on nutrients has a glow of scientific credibility, but in fact it has led consumers down an unhealthy road. When we view various foods simply as combinations of nutrients, we miss out on all kinds of other important information that goes into determining which foods are better choices for health and longevity. To someone who is just trying to "get my protein," there's no difference between a highly processed protein powder made from an isolated part of a soybean and the same amount of protein eaten in the form of whole beans. The all-important distinction between whole foods and processed foods is lost when we look at foods only as their nutrient components.

Furthermore, food companies shamelessly use nutrients as marketing slogans, proclaiming the presence of calcium, or protein, or fiber to give highly processed foods a "health halo" while hiding the sugar, fat, and refined flours in the small print on the label.

The focus on single nutrients obscures a critical truth: When it comes to food, the whole is greater than the sum of the parts. You could attempt to identify all the nutrients within a given food, a blueberry, for example, and put them into a pill, but it would never have the same healthy effects on your body as eating a bowl of blueberries. For a start, even the simplest food is more complex than we are currently capable of understanding in detail. And more importantly, even if we could know what all the parts are, that doesn't tell us how the whole works. Science has inadvertently shown this to be true, again and again, when it has attempted to isolate a particular nutrient and found that it behaves quite differently in the form of a pill than it does as part of a fruit or vegetable. One of the most dramatic examples involved the antioxidant beta-carotene, found in many fruits and vegetables. Studies showed that higher intake of beta-carotene-rich foods was associated with lower risk of death from certain cancers, but when beta-carotene was produced in a pill form, it appeared to actually increase the risk of mortality.[23]

The nutrients in your food interact with each other, with your body's unique biochemistry, and with the entire picture of your diet and lifestyle in far more intricate ways than science can yet comprehend. Foods are not merely collections of nutrients, any more than human beings are merely nutrient-processing systems. "Even the simplest food is a hopelessly complex thing to study," writes Pollan, "a virtual wilderness of chemical compounds, many of which exist in complex and dynamic relation to one another, and all of which together are in the process of changing from one state to another."[24] The good news, however, is that you don't necessarily need to understand it all if you simply *eat real food*. Your body will break it down into nutrients in the way it has evolved to do.

None of this is to say you should ignore the nutrients altogether—in fact, throughout this book we'll highlight some amazing nutrient properties of everyday whole foods and the powerful things they can do for your health. Our intention here is simply to encourage you to shift your focus first to *food* and to eat it in its whole form. Whole plant foods will supply the nutrients you need, both macro and micro, bundled together in beautifully evolved delivery systems that ensure you get maximum benefit.

Become a Whole Foodie

Imagine finding a way to eat that made you feel fantastic—nourished, vital, and satisfied. Ideally, it would be flexible enough to allow for your particular preferences but clear in its basic parameters. This diet would be simple enough to appeal to your common sense, and be backed by irrefutable science. You could just as easily explain it to your kids as you could defend it to your friends (even the most opinionated).

Now imagine being able to maintain a healthy weight without having to worry about portion sizes and never having to go on another crash diet. What if this way of eating could actually prevent common ailments; protect you from heart disease, cancer, and type 2 diabetes; and even reverse existing chronic conditions?

The Whole Foods Diet offers all of this and more. It's a sustainable, healthy way to eat and live. All of us authors and the many doctors, researchers, and dietitians featured in this book love food. We are foodies at heart, but not just any kind of foodie. We are *Whole Foodies*. A Whole Foodie loves great-tasting, life-enhancing food. And the best part is that food loves you right back—nourishing your body, empowering your immune system, and boosting your energy. Over the course of this book, we will explore all the many foods, meals, and dietary variations that one can enjoy as a Whole Foodie. From fans of the Mediterranean's bounty to passionate vegans to protein-loving Paleos, there are many different ways to embrace a whole foods, plant-based diet—with all the health benefits that naturally follow.

Today the options available for a Whole Foodie at just about any grocery store are simply unprecedented. Wonderful foods that will heal and revitalize our bodies call out to us, aisle after aisle. From all over the country and around the world, a paradise of fresh fruits and vegetables whispers its alluring message of health, vitality, and wellness. Nuts and seeds, hearty whole grains, healthy beans and other legumes, fresh-caught seafood, and pasture-raised animal foods are all within arm's reach.

Yet walk a few feet in the other direction, and the opposite is true. Cheap, seductive, easy-to-eat processed foods are all too readily available—foods that will, over time, break down our bodies and make us sick. Every day good people follow the siren song of sugar, fat, salt, and empty processed calories to a calamitous end. It may not hurt them today, and maybe not tomorrow, but eventually they suffer the unfortunate, often deadly consequences.

The choice you make, several times a day, to eat one type of food and not another, is the most important choice you could possibly make for your own health and longevity. The fact that you get to make it is a privilege, and also a great responsibility. A Whole Foodie embraces this choice gratefully and skillfully, choosing food that heals, food that nourishes, food that energizes, food that gives life. As long as you still eat every day, it's never too late to begin.

∽ WHOLE FOODIE TAKEAWAYS ∾

- **Become a skillful eater**—We have historically unprecedented food choices and nutritional knowledge available to us today. Challenge yourself to master the art of self-nourishment.
- **Eat real foods**—The first rule of any healthy diet is to choose unprocessed or whole foods and avoid highly processed and refined foods. Dr. Greger defines a whole food as one with "nothing bad added, nothing good taken away."
- **Eat more plants**—There is a wealth of evidence that those who eat more fruits, vegetables, legumes, and whole grains live longer and healthier lives and avoid chronic disease at higher rates. Aim to get 90% or more of your calories from the plant kingdom.

CHAPTER 2

Calorie Rich, Nutrient Poor

*Obesity, Chronic Disease, and the
Modern Dietary Dilemma*

"It is a hard matter, my fellow citizens,
to argue with the belly, since it has no ears."

—*Cato the Elder, Roman senator and historian*

For the first time in human history, obesity is a bigger health crisis globally than hunger. More people alive today will suffer disability as a result of consuming excess calories than as a result of consuming too few.[1] This stunning fact speaks volumes about the modern dietary dilemma. That's not to say hunger is no longer an issue in many areas of our planet, but it's striking that even in the developing world, a growing number of people now suffer the consequences of eating *too much* of the wrong kinds of food. And this shift has happened within the lifetimes of most people reading this book.

Overfed but undernourished, calorie rich but nutrient poor: this is the deadly paradox that has trapped hundreds of millions of human beings today. In America, where we created many of the eating patterns that are now being exported around the globe, the problem is especially acute. We've shared these statistics already, but they bear repeating: 69% of US adults are overweight; 36% are obese.[2] 17% of children are obese, and 19% have a diet-related chronic condition.[3] More than a million Americans die every year from heart disease and cancer, and more than 115 million are diabetic or prediabetic.[4]

The SAD Truth about American Diets

Since 1970, Americans' overall daily calorie intake has increased by a shocking 25%.[5] Unfortunately, those additional calories haven't come from healthy vegetables, the consumption of which actually went down by 3% in that time period (and keep in mind that "vegetables" in these surveys include French fries). Instead, the increased calories have come largely from added fats and oils (up 66%), dairy and dairy fats (up 18%), added fruit, largely in the form of fruit juice (up 25%), added sugars (up 10%), and added flour and cereal products (up 42%).[6] The Standard American Diet, often referred to by its apt acronym SAD, is not doing us any health favors. The average American gets about 54% of his or her calories from processed foods, 32% from animal products, and a paltry 14% from vegetables, fruits, nuts, beans, and whole grains.[7] Those statistics form both a disturbing pie chart and a recipe for chronically poor health.

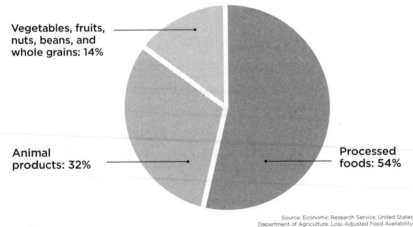

Vegetables, fruits, nuts, beans, and whole grains: 14%

Animal products: 32%

Processed foods: 54%

Source: Economic Research Service, United States Department of Agriculture: Loss-Adjusted Food Availability

As a result of these eating patterns, experts have lamented the fact that the generation being born today will very likely have a lower life expectancy than its parents, a first in American history. And even if life expectancy increases, what will be the quality of those added years? Consider that more people in this country are on prescription drugs than off.[8] We live in the age of chronic disease.

All of this bad news runs frustratingly counter to the story that modern

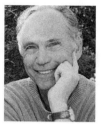

WHOLE FOODIE HERO
John Robbins

"The body has a remarkable capacity to begin healing itself, much more quickly than we had once thought possible."

Contributions: In 1987 Robbins published *Diet for a New America*, advocating a plant-based diet and highlighting the connections between food choices, environmentalism, and animal rights long before it was fashionable. The son of Baskin-Robbins Ice Cream cofounder Irv Robbins, he rejected his family's dairy legacy.

Fun facts: Whole Foodie passions run in the family. John and his son, Ocean Robbins, cofounded the popular Food Revolution Network, a movement committed to "healthy, sustainable, humane, and conscious food for all."

Read this: *The Food Revolution: How Your Diet Can Help Save Your Life and Our World*

Learn more: foodrevolution.org

medicine once told about its own potential. After all, wasn't this the institution that cured polio, reduced the infant mortality rate, created vaccines, and saved the lives of millions with antibiotics? Yes, and we all stand on the shoulders of those achievements. But in the last fifty years, the stakes have gone up. Our capacity to grow, process, and distribute food has exploded, while the best nutritional science is still struggling for a foothold in the medical mind. The "take a pill" attitude still dominates the medical and pharmaceutical industries.

Doctors today have little, if any, training in nutrition. "But wait a minute," the astute reader will say at this point. "Isn't it true that most deaths in the United States are related to diet and lifestyle?" Yes, and most chronic conditions as well. Surely it would be relevant for doctors to be well informed on that topic. Although medical schools could certainly do more to connect diet and disease, our point here is not to blame them; it is to appreciate the urgency of focusing more on diet and nutrition ourselves. Good information is out there; we just need to seek it out and apply it—in our grocery carts, in our kitchens, and at our dining room tables.

The Problem of Obesity

Human bodies come in all shapes and sizes, and so does beauty. Our intention is not to reinforce any particular social standard of attractiveness— this is a book about health and how what we eat can help us live longer, more vital lives. However, from a health perspective, there is an unavoidable connection between excess weight and a host of chronic conditions that all of us would much rather avoid.

Gaining weight is often the first warning sign that chronic disease is building up under the surface of your body. "Weight sits like a spider at the center of an intricate, tangled web of health and disease,"[9] writes Harvard Medical School's Dr. Willett. Strands in that web include heart disease, strokes, several types of cancer, diabetes, arthritis, and many more unpleasant and sometimes life-threatening conditions.[10] Maintaining a healthy body weight is therefore in our best interest if we want to remain vital, active, and glowing with the beauty that good health conveys for decades to come.

This is not to say that a healthy weight is a guarantee of health. If you're someone who maintains a lean body without much effort, you may think you're better off, but it's not necessarily true. You could still have heart disease, diabetes, or cancer developing in your body, even though you don't yet have a visible warning sign telling you how sick you are. I'm sure you've heard stories of the seemingly "thin and healthy" people who are suddenly struck down by diseases for which they didn't appear to be at risk.

Weight loss is a topic fraught with anxiety for many people. Too many of us have tried to lose weight, succeeded temporarily, and then fallen back. We've gone on endless diets, counted calories, controlled our portions, suffered feelings of deprivation, and struggled with the shame and self-hatred that often go with the territory. A whole foods, plant-based diet takes the drama out of downsizing, allowing you to reach and maintain your ideal weight and avoid the negative effects of caloric excess.

Craving Energy: Understanding Calorie Density

Several times a day, we each make the most critical choice we could possibly make for our own health and longevity. We choose to eat certain foods and in so doing we also choose not to eat others. We each have a daily caloric need, based on many factors ranging from our age and activity level to whether we are sick that day or did not eat enough the day before. (Government health recommendations estimate daily caloric needs to be 1,600 to 2,400 for adult women and 2,000 to 3,000 for adult men.) The type of calories we choose to consume to meet this need is up to us in any given moment.

So what is a calorie? A calorie is a measure of the energy contained in food. We all expend a certain amount of energy each day in order for our bodies to perform their functions. If we do any kind of physical exercise, manual labor, or other activity, we expend some more. The food we eat is a fuel source that provides us with that energy. Calories come in three forms: carbohydrates, fat, and protein. If we consume more energy than we expend, the body will store the excess energy in the form of fat and we will gain weight. If we consume less, our bodies will need other sources of fuel, burning stored fat and leading to weight loss.

Different types of food contain vastly different amounts of calories relative to their weights. If you take one pound of lettuce and compare it to one pound of cheese, for example, the lettuce has far fewer calories than the cheese. The cheese, therefore, is more "calorie dense."

For hundreds of thousands of years, the main problem human beings and their evolutionary predecessors faced was getting enough calories to stay alive. The less time we spent gathering food the better, because that reduced the risk of falling prey to wild animals. Therefore, we evolved to seek out the

What Does Two Hundred Calories Look Like?

A full plate of mixed steamed vegetables (four cups)

One very large baked sweet potato

A small bowl (one cup) of black bean soup

Four chicken nuggets

Three-quarters of a glazed donut

Three one-inch cubes of cheese

Two tablespoons of olive oil

foods that would give us more calories to less bulk; in other words, the most calorie-dense foods (see chapter 11 for more on why). Cheese wasn't on the menu back in our hunter-gatherer days, but our ancestors would have been drawn to the more calorie-dense fruits and vegetables—for example, they might have chosen wild nuts over wild greens. And when they could get it, the occasional piece of wild lean meat would have been attractive.

This equation worked fairly well for most of human history. As long as we were choosing between whole plant foods, with the occasional addition of lean meat, our attraction to the most calorie-dense options did not present a problem when it came to maintaining a healthy weight. Indeed, it was essential for staying alive. Of course, the less-calorie-dense foods contain important nutrients, and evolution has ensured that their variety of delicious tastes and textures keeps us coming back for those as well. But there was little chance of our eating too many calories, because the amount of bulk we needed to consume in order to meet our needs would fill us up.

The Feeling of Fullness: Understanding Satiety

Weight loss gurus are fond of reducing the process to a simple formula: calories in < calories out. So long as you consume fewer calories than you expend, you'll lose weight. Makes sense, in theory. But in order to make this formula work for you in practice, you need to understand that not all calories are created equal when it comes to filling you up. Some come in the form of fiber-rich, nutrient-rich foods that will leave you feeling full and satisfied. Others come in the form of refined, fiber-stripped, highly processed foods that contain few or no nutrients and will leave you hungry, making you more likely to eat more. A chicken nugget is so calorie dense that after eating only two, you've consumed a hundred calories, the equivalent of a whole bowl of lentil soup (one and a quarter cups). And who stops at two chicken nuggets? You'll probably want to eat at least ten, or twelve, taking in five or six hundred calories very quickly. With the lentil soup, by comparison, you'll probably feel full after just one bowl, or maybe two. To lose weight, or to maintain a healthy weight, the key is to choose foods that give you adequate calories but not too many, while making you feel full so that you're less likely to overeat.

There's a term for the feeling of fullness: *satiety*. It's a physical sensation that is the opposite of hunger. Just as hunger is the body's mechanism for telling you to eat, satiety is the body's mechanism for telling you to stop. Unfortunately, food processing has wreaked havoc with these instincts so that many of us can no longer trust the signals our bodies are giving us. As long as we are eating highly processed, refined foods, we are likely to feel hungry even when we've eaten more calories than we need, and we won't experience satiety until we've overeaten.

Here's what we know about how satiety works. There are "receptors" in the stomach and digestive tract that measure the food we ingest in several ways. One thing they measure is the weight and bulk of the food, or the amount of "stretch" that occurs in the stomach to make room for the food. This is why foods containing a lot of fiber fill us up more—they take up more space and trigger a signal to the brain that says enough has been eaten. Foods that have been refined and processed (with fiber and water removed) take up less space, so even though they contain more calories, the message does not get back to your brain that you've had enough.

You also have "receptors" that ensure you are consuming calories and not just getting stretch without caloric content. When you're eating whole plant foods, these tend to work quite accurately, together with the stretch receptors, to ensure that you get the right amount of food and not too much. Over the last few decades, however, the rise of processed food has fundamentally altered this algorithm. Processing tends to increase the calorie density of any given food by:

• removing water
• reducing or removing fiber
• adding sugar and/or fat.

As we alter our food in this way, its bulk/weight decreases (because of the removal of fiber and water) and the number of calories increases (due to added fat and/or sugar). Hence the number of calories relative to weight increases dramatically. For example, corn, which contains 500 calories per pound, becomes corn oil, at 4,000 calories per pound. A sweet potato, which weighs in at 389 calories per pound, gets cut up and deep-fried in that oil to become sweet potato chips, at 2,400 calories per pound. Beets, at just 200 calories per pound, become refined sugar, at 1,800 calories per pound.

When you eat these unnaturally concentrated foods, your calorie receptors and stretch receptors no longer correlate. You're getting a lot of calories, but very little bulk. With its two measurement systems out of sync, your body is confused. The message that goes back to the brain reads something like this: "I think we got enough calories, but maybe I am wrong, because I don't feel full." So we eat more to fill our stomachs, and in the process we overconsume calories. The problem gets exaggerated when the calories come in liquid form, as with oils, juices, or sugary drinks, which stretch the stomach barely if at all, but contain a lot of calories. This is why one of the most important pieces of weight-loss advice you'll ever hear is, *Don't drink your calories!*

Those extra calories accumulate over time. Three thousand five hundred additional calories equals one additional pound of fat, so if you overshoot your needs by as little as one hundred calories a meal (two chicken nuggets) and you do this three times a day, you will gain a pound of fat every two weeks, which adds up to more than twenty-five pounds in a year.

It's not only processed foods that mess with our satiety signals. Animal foods also lack fiber while being calorie dense. Today's factory-farmed, grain-fed animals bear little resemblance to the lean wild game that our ancestors might have feasted on after an occasional hunt. When we eat their meats, cooked in oil, alongside other calorie-dense, fiber-deficient foods like white bread, fries, ketchup, and so on, it's a recipe for obesity.

Now that these foods are part of our everyday menu of choices, our evolutionary propensity to choose the most calorie-dense options has become a problem. We are no longer choosing between lettuce and a banana; we are choosing between a banana and a burger, and the evolutionary mechanism that kept our ancestors well fueled is leading us down a dangerous path.

When we choose the burger, and pair it with an order of fries and a soda, we get more than a thousand calories in a single sitting. Fast food is not just ready in minutes—it's eaten and digested equally quickly because it has already been refined and broken down, requiring astonishingly little effort to consume.

Why Diets Don't Work

Once you understand the basic principles of calorie density and satiety, you can start to make sense of why so many people find their weight creeping up. It also clarifies why dieting, which relies on portion control and calorie restriction, rarely works. It's not because you lack self-control or willpower; it's because the environment in which you live is making foods available to you that subvert your body's natural instincts and trick you into feeling hungry when you've already consumed more calories than you need.

Hunger is a powerful survival mechanism, and it is very hard to defeat it through willpower alone. After all, your brain thinks that the lack of stretch

The Veggie Paradox

Would you like to know how to lose weight without having to give up anything? Here's the secret: Eat *more* vegetables! Add at least one extra serving of veggies (or fruits) to what you would normally eat at each meal, and be sure to eat those before anything else, and you'll discover the veggie paradox— the more veggies you eat, the more weight you lose (assuming you don't cover those veggies in fatty dressings or sauces or cook them in oils).

When you eat whole fruits and veggies, you fill yourself up with low-calorie, fiber-rich, nutrient-rich foods that will leave you less hungry for processed foods or animal foods. A good strategy is to start every meal with a big salad or a bowl of vegetable soup (or a bowl of fruit, if you prefer, at breakfast).

Eat more veggies and lose more weight—that's the beauty of the veggie paradox!

means you are actually calorie deficient and starving, so it continues sending hunger signals in an attempt to keep you alive. Sooner or later you're likely to respond to it by eating more.

The good news is that by choosing whole foods, mostly plants, you can begin to trust your own body again. You won't have to obsessively monitor your portion sizes or deny your hunger; in fact, you may have to retrain yourself to eat larger meals than you are accustomed to if you have been in the habit of controlling portions to manage your weight. These are the foods your body thrives on, and they also happen to be the foods that your body can measure accurately, because they correlate calorie density and stretch. Your satiety signals will become more trustworthy as you choose foods that are naturally nutritious and filling.

Eating whole foods, mostly plants, is a great recipe for sustained weight loss because they combine high fiber and water content with low calorie density. However, for it to work, you need to make sure you eat enough.

That's right, *eat enough*! This is not a diet of portion control or deprivation. If you choose only the foods that are lowest in calorie density, you'll continue to feel hungry. Therefore, it's important to also eat highly satiating plant foods like starchy vegetables (yams, squash, corn, potatoes, and so on), whole grains (rice, wheat, oats, and so on), and legumes (beans, peas, lentils, and so on) to ensure that you meet your energy needs without having to consume mountains of food to simply get enough calories. Combining fresh vegetables and fruits with whole grains, legumes, and starchy vegetables is the best mix to ensure that you'll feel full *and* lose excess weight.

Studies have confirmed the important relationships between calorie density, satiety, and overconsumption. Subjects in these studies are divided into two groups, one eating a calorie-dense diet and the other eating a less calorie-dense diet. They are allowed to eat when hungry until they are full. The results are clear: those fed high-calorie-density diets tend to take in more calories and gain weight, while those fed lower-calorie-density diets tend to take in fewer calories (even though they consume more bulk) and lose weight. One such study concluded, "Our findings support the hypothesis that a relation exists between the consumption of an energy-dense diet and obesity and provide evidence of the importance of fruit and vegetable consumption for weight management."[11]

Choose a whole foods, plant-based diet, and you will quickly be on your way toward reaching and maintaining your ideal weight. However, this is not simply a weight-loss book, and the Whole Foods Diet offers much more than a trim waist. Our goal is to help you learn to eat for optimum health and use diet to prevent or reverse disease. In order to do this, there is another key principle you need to understand.

Nutrient Density: Making Every Calorie Count

The concept of "nutrient density" has been reinvented and popularized by Joel Fuhrman, MD, one of the most important thinkers and practitioners in modern nutrition, and it is at the heart of his popular "Nutritarian" approach to eating (not to be confused with Pollan's "nutritionism," discussed on page 40). Dr. Fuhrman explains this idea with a formula:

$$\text{Health} = \text{Nutrients/Calories}$$

In other words, to be healthy, you need to choose foods that grant you a favorable amount of nutrients per calorie. That's what *nutrient dense* means. When Fuhrman talks about nutrients, he's not referring to the macronutrients— protein, fats, and carbohydrates—the elements in our food that deliver calories. He's referring to what he calls "noncaloric food factors," or micronutrients— including vitamins, minerals, fiber, and phytochemicals. Some foods contain a lot of calories but few or even no nutrients, in this sense. Fuhrman's approach to eating is to "make every calorie count"[13] by striving to get an adequate amount and diversity of micronutrients from our food every day.

What Are Micronutrients?

Micronutrient is a general term describing essential dietary elements that are not sources of calories, but that the human body requires in small quantities. These include vitamins, minerals, and phytochemicals. You're probably familiar with those first two categories, but what are phytochemicals? These are a more recently discovered type of micronutrient. *Phyto* means plant, and phytochemicals are biologically active compounds found in plants. There are believed to be as many as four thousand different phytochemicals, though many have not yet been identified. They have various functions, but many appear to be powerful protectors against disease and supporters of immune function.

Dr. Fuhrman writes that these micronutrients provide "a secondary level of nutrition that adds a complex layer of disease resistance and longevity benefits."[12] While the complex world of phytochemicals and their interactions with the human body is only beginning to be explored, what we already know is reason enough to eat a wide variety of fruits and vegetables.

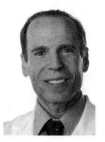

WHOLE FOODIE HERO
Joel Fuhrman, MD

"There is no magic...no miracle weight-loss pill. There is only the natural world of law and order, of cause and effect. If you want optimal health and longevity, you must engage the cause. And if you want to lose fat weight safely, you must eat a diet of predominantly unrefined foods that are nutrient- and fiber-rich."

Contributions: Dr. Fuhrman's reinvention of the concept of nutrient density has changed the way many people relate to fruits and vegetables. His Nutritarian diet, popularized in his numerous books and PBS shows, has inspired thousands to transform their health and reverse disease.

Fun facts: Dr. Fuhrman was once a world-class figure skater and would likely have competed at the 1976 Olympics had it not been for a career-stopping heel injury, which turned out to be the unexpected doorway to his career as a doctor.

Read this: *Eat to Live: The Amazing Nutrient-Rich Program for Fast and Sustained Weight Loss*

Learn More: DrFuhrman.com

This may sound like a commonsense idea, but it leads to quite a radical reevaluation of foods. If you were to ask the average American what foods contain the most nutrients, he or she would probably rank meats like beef and chicken pretty high, having been raised to consider "protein" the most important element of nutrition. And yet by Fuhrman's measure, leafy greens like kale and romaine far outrank meats on the nutrient density scale. Have you ever wondered why kale suddenly became such a popular health food a few years back? It was partly due to Fuhrman, who awarded this rather tough leafy green the top score in his ANDI (Aggregate Nutrient Density Index) system for measuring nutrient density, a perfect 1,000. When Whole Foods Market started using his system in stores, sales of kale skyrocketed.

MY WHOLE FOODIE STORY

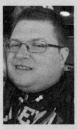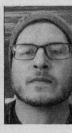

Russell Cartwright, 42, Annapolis, Maryland

At twenty-one, I weighed 314 pounds. I successfully lost weight, but not in a very healthy way. By the time I turned thirty, I'd gained it all back, and this time I couldn't shift it. I assumed my metabolism had just slowed down.

One day I went to increase my life insurance policy, and they gave me a whole list of bad news. I was type 2 diabetic, my blood sugar level was extremely high, and my cholesterol was through the roof. I was scared, really scared.

I knew I had to change what I ate, but I didn't know how. I was a burgers-pizza-and-beer kind of guy, but I just made the effort to start eating more fruits and vegetables and I lost my first twenty-five pounds. Then I was offered the opportunity to attend Dr. Joel Fuhrman's Immersion through my job at Whole Foods—and that's what really changed my life.

I lost 116 pounds in one year, and got off my diabetes medicine. My blood sugar levels are now normal and my cholesterol level is really good.

These days I eat lots of fruits and vegetables, and I have a huge salad every dinner. I don't eat 100% plant-based—I'll sometimes add chicken to my salad, though I don't eat red meat. I never eat fast food, ever. I eat broccoli and hummus, religiously—that's my favorite. I eat foods I'd never tasted before, like avocados.

It really helped me to document what I ate, and to ask my team leaders at Whole Foods Market to hold me accountable. That was crucial. I decided to approach my health with the same attitude I brought to my professional life. I also started working out and discovered that I really enjoy that part of my day.

I never called it a diet. I'm not rigid about it. If I'm traveling one day and I eat something less healthy, I don't make a big deal out of it—I just get right back to the healthy stuff the next day. I tell my friends, "Don't call it a diet. Just change what you eat." It saved me.

Kale (like other dark green leafy cruciferous vegetables) is packed with phytochemicals and fiber but low in calories; hence it has an extraordinarily high ratio of nutrients to calories. As Fuhrman is fond of pointing out, in his lectures and often on his T-shirt, "Kale is the new beef!"

Dr. Fuhrman is outspoken about the misinformation that runs rampant in the diet world. One topic he's particularly passionate about is metabolism. "Nutritional scientists the world over recognize that excess calories reduce our life span, while lower caloric intake extends life span," he declares. "And yet people all over America are trying to use fads and tricks to *speed up* their metabolic rates so they can eat more calories without getting fat. That doesn't make any sense! By speeding up your metabolism, you're aging yourself!"[14]

Dr. Fuhrman's Aggregate Nutrient Density Index (ANDI)

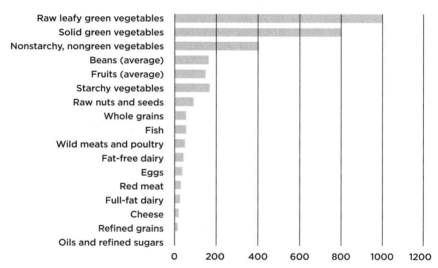

Fuhrman's concept of nutrient density is a powerful tool for shifting your focus away from what you *shouldn't* eat and toward all the wonderful foods you *should* eat in order to maximize your nutrients. But before you rush out armed with an ANDI chart to start measuring one vegetable against another, it's important to understand that compared to processed foods and animal foods, *all natural plant foods are nutrient dense.* The most important thing is that you eat plenty of them, and if broccoli doesn't score

A Note about Exercise

This book is focused on health and diet. However, another important element of lifestyle change, particularly if you are trying to lose weight, is exercise. While a whole foods, plant-based diet enables weight loss even without exercise, regular exercise will only enhance its benefits. Exercise has been shown to improve cardiovascular health, reduce blood sugar, improve bone health, and increase one's overall sense of well-being, and it may even increase satiety and suppress the desire to overeat.[15]

Even a short daily walk is better than no exercise at all. If you don't like going to the gym, look for activities you can build into your day that improve your strength, balance, flexibility, and endurance. One of the hallmarks of the longest-lived cultures in the world (see chapter 4) is that they all engage in "natural movement"—walking, gardening, getting up and down from the floor, herding goats in hilly terrain. They are not necessarily lifting weights at the gym, but they are keeping their bodies strong and flexible.

One benefit of eating a whole foods, plant-based diet is that it will give you more energy for exercising. Perhaps you'll awaken a new love for hiking, running, tennis, or yoga as you shed excess weight and feel better in your body.

If you're already active, this way of eating will only enhance your performance. A whole foods, plant-based diet improves your cardiovascular system, boosts your power, and speeds up your recovery rate.[16] Some people fear that they'll lose strength without large amounts of animal protein, but the many plant-based athletes out there—from Olympian track and field medalist Carl Lewis to tennis superstars Venus Williams and Novak Djokovic to ultra-athletes Rich Roll and Scott Jurek—are testimony that this is not the case.

quite as high as collard greens, that's no reason to stop eating it. If you simply eat a whole foods, plant-based diet and include a wide variety of fruits and vegetables, you will naturally be getting a much higher amount of nutrients per calorie than anyone who eats a diet heavy in processed foods and animal foods.

Don't pass over the plant foods that rank lower on the ANDI scale, like nuts, seeds, starchy vegetables, whole grains, legumes, and fresh fruit. These still contain plenty of beneficial nutrients. Dr. Fuhrman does not recommend a diet of only eating the highest ANDI scoring foods such as leafy greens. These foods are important to include, but he also recommends a diversity of other plant foods for excellent health, protection against cancer, and longevity. In fact, fruits, beans, and seeds are an important part of his healthful program.

Nutrient density. Calorie density. Satiety. These are all critical concepts to understand, enabling you to choose foods that ensure you'll be well nourished *and* well satisfied.

꩜ WHOLE FOODIE TAKEAWAYS ꩜

• **Understand calorie density**—Human beings have an evolutionary predilection to seek out the most calorie-dense foods. Highly processed foods are extremely calorie dense but lack the bulk to stretch the stomach, therefore confusing the body's natural systems to know when to stop eating. Choose fiber-rich whole plant foods and you can trust your body to tell you when you've had enough.
• **Eat a variety of fruits and veggies**—Plant foods are packed with health-promoting, disease-fighting nutrients. Per calorie, they are far more nutrient dense than animal foods. Eat lots of different fruits and vegetables, as well as legumes and whole grains, to maximize these benefits.

CHAPTER 3

Connecting Diet and Disease

Nutritional Science Looks at the Big Picture

"To understand is to perceive patterns."

—*Isaiah Berlin, The Proper Study of Mankind: An Anthology of Essays*

Consider this scenario for a moment. If someone offered you a pill that had been shown to prevent and reverse heart disease and type 2 diabetes; lower cholesterol, blood pressure, and body weight; significantly reduce your risk of getting multiple types of cancer; extend your life span; and make you look and feel great, would you hesitate to take it? It may not come in a bottle, but, as you will see in this book, a whole foods, plant-based diet has been shown to do all these things.

On the other hand, consider the following scientific findings. High consumption of red meat and processed meats has been connected with greater risk of death from all causes, including chronic diseases such as cardiovascular disease and type 2 diabetes.[1] Eating large amounts of animal protein has been correlated with higher incidences of cancer[2] and mortality.[3] More than a thousand studies on bowel cancer risk have confirmed that red meat increases risk while high-fiber plant foods decrease it.[4] Processed meats are particularly scary, with significant studies linking them to stomach cancer, breast cancer, and colon cancer, and the World Health Organization classifying them as a carcinogen.[5] As a result, the World Cancer Research Fund International and the American Institute for Cancer Research came out with firm recommendations for people to "eat mostly foods of plant origin,"[6] including whole grains, fruits, vegetables, and beans.

Varieties of Nutritional Science

Nutritional science comes in many forms. Here are a few common types of study:

Epidemiological studies, observational studies, and cohort studies are big-picture approaches in which researchers examine one or more populations (or cohorts) of people over time, noting their health outcomes, their diets, and various other lifestyle factors, and comparing them to other populations.

Randomized controlled trials (RCTs) are clinical trials in which participants are randomly assigned to two or more groups, one of which is a control group, which receives no actual treatment. (For example, in a drug trial, those in this group might receive a sugar pill.) This format means that experimenters are better able to rule out factors other than the one being studied.

Laboratory trials involve testing specific nutrients or supplements on tissue samples, animals, or humans and observing the results over time.

Meta-analyses compare multiple studies done on similar subjects and draw out common themes.

Each of these approaches has strengths and weaknesses. In the end, we need many different kinds of science to help us get the best picture of the relationship between health and diet.

These studies are not simply outliers. In fact, they are just a few among a multitude of compelling data points that make the case for a whole foods, plant-based diet. The research supporting the wisdom of this way of eating, even briefly summarized, is enough to fill several books. Rigorous laboratory experiments, carefully controlled clinical trials, and long-term observational studies following millions of people over several decades confirm the profound value of eating more real plant-based foods and minimizing highly processed foods and animal products.

Challenging American Dietary Dogma: The China Study

Scientists have various methods at their disposal when it comes to studying diet, health, and longevity. They can study a population of healthy people, perform controlled studies on two groups eating different diets, or isolate nutrients for examination in the laboratory. Any of these approaches could be called "nutritional science," but they are so distinct that they might as well be different fields. Some look at the big picture, seeking patterns and trends; others focus on detailed, specific chemical processes. Each method offers valid and important insights into the riddle of health, and each also has its limitations and blind spots. While most scientists stake their entire careers on one particular type of research, occasionally you meet a rare inquirer whose quest for knowledge has included both the macro and the micro, the big picture and the isolated details. T. Colin Campbell is one such man.

If the field of nutrition had an aristocracy, Campbell would surely be part of it. He may not have been the first to demonstrate significant connections between diet and disease, but he did so on a scale that was unmatched. His career-defining work was known as The China Study (or The China-Cornell-Oxford Project, to give it its full title)—a massive twenty-year epidemiological study that examined the eating habits and diseases of 6,500 people in sixty-five Chinese provinces. A 1990 *New York Times* article called it "the most comprehensive large study ever undertaken of the relationship between diet and the risk of developing disease" and reported that even its early findings were "challenging much of American dietary dogma."[7]

What were Campbell's controversial findings? He sums up the essential message this way: "People who ate the most animal-based foods got the most chronic disease. . . . People who ate the most plant-based foods were the healthiest and tended to avoid chronic disease."[8]

Campbell would once have seemed an unlikely candidate to become an advocate for plant-based eating. Growing up on a dairy farm in the beautiful Virginia countryside, the young Campbell believed that "the good old American diet is the best there is. The more dairy, meat, and eggs we

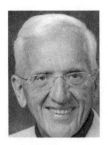

WHOLE FOODIE HERO
T. Colin Campbell, MD

"At this point, any scientist, doctor, journalist, or policy maker who denies or minimizes the importance of a whole food, plant-based diet for individual and societal well-being simply isn't looking clearly at the facts. There's just too much good evidence to ignore anymore."

Contributions: Pioneering the science of plant-based eating. As Dr. Dean Ornish puts it: "Everyone in the field of nutrition science stands on the shoulders of Dr. Campbell."

Fun facts: Campbell coined the term "whole food, plant-based," using it way back in 1978.

Read this: *The China Study: The Most Comprehensive Study of Nutrition Ever Conducted*

Learn more: nutritionstudies.org

consumed, the better."[9] After studying at Penn State, Cornell, and MIT, and teaching at Virginia Tech, he returned to Cornell as a professor in 1975. He helped set nutritional policy guidelines, provided information for and sat on governmental committees, generated key original research funded by top institutions, set standards for health programs, and developed policy for international food and nutrition programs. And yet, even as he ascended to the top of the health and nutrition establishment, he was beginning to question its tenets.

Campbell slowly began to suspect that the meat- and dairy-heavy American diet was playing a significant role in the epidemics of heart disease, cancer, and diabetes. By the late 1970s, he had shown strong evidence in his laboratory that certain nutrients, including proteins derived from animal-based foods, were involved in promoting the development of cancerous tumors in animals. Plant-based foods, on the other hand, seemed to be a factor in decreasing tumor development. These studies, however, were limited to animals, and they focused on specific, isolated nutrients in carefully controlled circumstances. "Nutrient by nutrient. That's the way we did research, that's the way I taught it,"[10] Campbell says. And this form of research has its limits. Each nutrient interacts with other nutrients in a thousand different ways, and the more we seek to isolate one and vigilantly rule out all these various interdependent relationships, the more we distance ourselves from nutrition in the real world. As Campbell told the *New York Times,* "I came to believe…that there was a very different world of understanding nutrition. We shouldn't be thinking in a linear way that A causes B. We should be thinking about how things work together."[11] And to be able to study how things worked together, he needed to follow a large population over a long period of time.

Around this time, Campbell met a Chinese scientist, Dr. Chen Junshi, who would provide just that opportunity. Junshi told Campbell that in the early 1970s, Zhou Enlai, premier of the People's Republic of China, had been dying of cancer and had initiated the China Health and Nutrition Survey, the largest survey of its kind ever completed.

The survey—which had collected data from 880 million Chinese citizens, or 96% of the population—showed fascinating patterns. Cancer rates, it revealed, were often geographic in nature. In some rural areas there was little or no evidence of the disease, while other regions, particularly urban ones, showed dramatic increases. Inspired by the breadth of this data, Campbell and Junshi proposed an extensive survey of dietary and lifestyle habits.

Late-twentieth-century China offered a uniquely fertile ground for a study of diet and disease. The population was genetically very similar, but varied significantly in dietary habits, disease rates, and other environmental factors from region to region. In sixty-five rural and semirural regions of China, Campbell and his team administered questionnaires, took blood and urine samples, analyzed foods from local markets, and carefully measured participating families' food intake over a period of a few days. "When we were done," Campbell writes, "we had more than 8,000 statistically

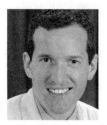

WHOLE FOODIE HERO
Thomas Campbell, MD

"The food you eat is so profoundly instrumental to your health that breakfast, lunch, and dinner are in fact exercises in medical decision-making."

Contributions: Thomas Campbell, coauthor of *The China Study*, is a pioneering plant-based physician in his own right. He is clinical director of the Program for Nutrition at the University of Rochester Medical Center, the first program of its kind to focus on the health value of a whole foods, plant-based diet.

Fun facts: Dr. Campbell's first career choice was not medicine or nutrition, but acting. He was struggling to make a name for himself in Chicago when his father asked him to help with the writing of *The China Study*. He agreed, and within a few years was not only a best-selling author but also had earned a medical degree and completed his physician training.

Read this: *The China Study Solution: The Simple Way to Lose Weight and Reverse Illness, Using a Whole-Food, Plant-Based Diet*

Learn more: nutritionstudies.org

significant associations between lifestyle, diet, and disease variables."[12]

What did The China Study show? It conclusively demonstrated that the regions in which people ate the most animal products, which tended to be the wealthiest regions, had the highest rates of heart disease, cancer, and other chronic degenerative diseases, leading Campbell to call them "diseases of affluence." In contrast, in the regions of greater poverty, people ate fewer animal foods and had lower rates of these diseases.

What specifically caused these diseases of affluence? Was it the saturated fat found in animal foods? Was it animal protein itself or a particular type of animal meat? Was it dietary cholesterol, which is found only in animal foods? These are questions that were beyond the scope of Campbell's

Fiber Is Your Friend

One key finding of The China Study is the association of a high-fiber diet with a decrease in certain cancers, including colon cancer. Chinese consumption of dietary fiber averaged three times what is typically found in American diets.

Fiber is a critical component of a whole foods, plant-based diet. It is the substance that gives structure to the cell walls of plants in the same way that bones give structure to the bodies of animals. Because of this, high fiber intake is one of the markers of a plant-heavy diet.

Fiber was once thought to be an unnecessary addition to the human diet. After all, we digest very little if any of it. But recent years have seen a new appreciation of its importance, confirming the findings of earlier researchers, including T. Colin Campbell and Denis Burkitt. It turns out that fiber plays a critical role in feeding our good gut bacteria. We may not digest it, but they do! It also performs a cleansing, or "scrubbing," function. Fiber makes everything work better and move better as well. It improves digestion, stabilizes blood sugar levels, detoxifies, keeps our pH low, and helps with the excretion of unwanted substances from the body.

Today the Standard American Diet is largely deficient in fiber, weighing in at around fifteen grams per day. That's not enough. And put down the Metamucil—there is good evidence that merely adding fiber as a supplement does not bring with it the same health benefits. Your body needs the real thing—which only comes in whole plant foods such as fruits, vegetables, legumes, beans, and whole grains.

research. Still, it's impossible not to notice the striking relationships between higher consumption of animal products, the adoption of more Western-style diets, and higher rates of obesity, heart disease, cancer, and diabetes.

For those championing the health potential of whole foods, plant-based diets, The China Study has become an important touchstone. The book, written by Campbell and his son, Thomas Campbell, MD, was published in 2005, and has shocked the publishing world by selling close to two million copies. But the epidemiological approach to nutrition (see box, page 64) is not without its critics, many of whom don't like this type of "observational" research. They claim that such studies cannot easily isolate particular foods or nutrients or assign clear causal links between a certain food and a certain outcome. They cannot eliminate other factors that might be playing a role, such as environmental conditions. They draw correlations and reveal patterns and trends, but correlation, as is often said, does not equal causation. Of course, it should be said that T. Colin Campbell, who has done every kind of nutritional research, is well aware of the scope and limitations of observational data.

Such criticisms are often combined with an insistence that randomized controlled trials (see box, page 64) are the only surefire means of resolving nutritional questions. We beg to differ. While RCTs are useful for testing drugs, their downside—and it's a significant one—is that they do not easily lend themselves to the study of long-term dietary effects. The types of chronic disease that are diet related, such as heart disease and cancer, tend to develop slowly, over years and even decades. The much shorter time frames of more controlled studies (measured in months instead of years and decades) are often not sufficient to show the results that really matter. Furthermore, it is almost impossible to randomize people to follow specific diets over a long period, and often not ethically acceptable to do so, just as it was not acceptable to force nonsmokers to smoke for thirty years to determine "definitively" whether smoking was harmful. We would do well to remember that the evidence for the relationship between smoking and cancer came from epidemiological studies, and the tobacco industry used the "correlation is not causation" argument for years as a key weapon in its arsenal of rebuttals.

"The Healthiest People in the World"

The data from The China Study is extremely compelling, but are there other studies that have come to similar conclusions, ones that have been conducted a little closer to home? The answer is yes. One such group of studies has been derived from a unique population of Americans, the Seventh-day Adventists, a Christian religious sect established in the mid-nineteenth century. Many of the Adventists are inspired by the biblical verse Genesis 1:29: "And God said, Behold, I have given you every herb bearing seed, which *is* upon the face of all the earth, and every tree, in the which *is* the fruit of a tree yielding seed; to you it shall be for meat." In other words, eat real foods, mostly plants.

The Adventists are one of the most interesting groups to study, from the perspective of diet, because they have such a similar overall lifestyle (some distinguishing factors being that there are very few smokers or alcohol consumers, they have a strong religious faith and community, and they exercise regularly), but at the same time, specific members follow different dietary patterns. These range from vegan (no animal products) to lacto-ovo vegetarian (vegetarian with dairy and eggs), to pesco-vegetarian (vegetarian with some fish) to meat-eaters. It is rare in epidemiological studies that researchers can observe a group of people with very similar lifestyles but so many distinct dietary subgroups, enabling them to more effectively isolate the impact of diet on health.

In the first Adventist study, conducted in the 1970s and '80s in California, more than thirty-four thousand people were followed for fourteen years.[13] The first thing that jumps out about the data is that the Adventists who ate a *primarily* plant-based diet—the vegans, lacto-ovo vegetarians, and pesco-vegetarians (collectively referred to by researchers as "the vegetarians")—were the longest-lived populations, not just among their fellow Adventists, but among all Californians, and possibly in the world! In fact, Loma Linda, California—where there is a large community of Adventists—has been identified as one of the world's five longevity hot spots, the "Blue Zones," which we will discuss in chapter 4. For now, let us just say that the Adventists have a life span worth studying—the vegetarian men and women live to be about eighty-three and eighty-six, respectively (compared to seventy-six and eighty-one for the average American).[14] And if you just look at those who also had healthy lifestyles, meaning no smoking, regular exercising, and so on, the average life span jumps to eighty-seven and ninety. That is an extra eleven years of life for men and nine for women!

When it comes to America's leading causes of death—heart disease and cancer—the vegetarian Adventists again fare well. They have the lowest rate of heart disease in the nation.[15] In men, the risk of fatal heart disease was "significantly related to beef intake."[16] The risk of colon cancer was increased by 88% in Adventists who ate meat over their vegetarian counterparts. Diabetes, our rapidly growing national epidemic, is rare among the Adventists. Indeed, they boast the nation's lowest rates of the disease.[17]

Part of what make the Adventist Health Studies so remarkable is the geographical context of the population. For example, Loma Linda, California,

Five Tips for Digesting Nutritional Science

We don't all have time to become experts in nutritional science, so it's understandable we turn to the popular media for bite-size, predigested versions. However, when it comes to something as important as what you eat, we encourage you to take a few extra steps to ensure you entrust your health to reliable sources of information.

1. Go to the Source
Don't get fooled by a dramatic headline. Read the substance of the story and, if necessary, check out the actual study. You might be surprised how different they can be.

2. Ask Who's Behind It
Unfortunately, too many food companies are initiating, funding, and even writing up the studies that make their products look good. A shocking percentage of studies published in leading medical journals are commercially funded.[18] Of course, funding conflicts of interest don't always indicate bad science, but never underestimate how simple it can be to design studies that obtain results favorable to particular interest groups.

is hardly tucked away on an isolated island, cut off from contemporary society's dietary habits. No, it is right in the middle of southern California's cultural melting pot, just south of the San Bernardino freeway. In other words, they live among us. And yet, healthwise, they might as well exist on a different planet. Indeed, their health outcomes are like a bright shining vision of possibility in the midst of America's chronic disease dystopia.

In 2002 a second major Adventist study was started, led by Dr. Gary Fraser and a team of researchers from Loma Linda University, which included ninety-six thousand participants from across the United States and Canada. The results from that study showed that Adventist meat-eaters had the biggest waistlines, and had a higher death rate than their vegetarian Adventist counterparts. They also tended to have worse overall dietary

3. Consider How Well It Is Designed

The devil is often in the details, and study design matters. Is butter good for you? If you design a study that compares it to margarine, the result may tell you more about the deficiency of margarine than the ultimate nutritional value of butter. Journalists regularly fall for this kind of thing, especially if it allows them to write a surprising or "shocking" headline.

4. Look for Backup

When it comes to nutrition, single studies must be looked at in light of larger trends. Are there corroborating studies? Don't take any single study too seriously if it is only one of many on the subject; give the most credence to general trends. If a hundred studies implicate refined sugars in health troubles, and two outliers exonerate them, don't use that as a justification to order dessert.

5. Find Trusted Sources

This final tip may be the most important. Very few of us have the time or expertise to research nutrition by ourselves. We must rely on trusted sources to give us the straight scoop. All the Whole Foodie Heroes we feature in this book have websites and books that you may find helpful in your quest for better health.

habits, including greater consumption of highly processed foods such as sugar, soda, and refined grains. This raises the question of whether it was the animal foods or the processed foods or both that led to shorter lives in this cohort. Although we cannot tease that out with this study, what we can tell is that the lacto-ovo vegetarians, the pesco-vegetarians, and the vegans all had significantly lower mortality rates compared to the meat-eaters.[19]

A similar pattern was observed with type 2 diabetes—prevalence of the disease increased from the vegans at the low end (2.6%) to the lacto-ovo vegetarians (3.2%) to the pesco-vegetarians (4.8%) to the meat-eaters (7.6%)[20]

It's worth noting that even those Adventists classified as meat-eaters were much less so than most Americans. The meat-eating Adventists' diet (in terms of daily intake in grams) was largely composed of fruits and vegetables, nuts, legumes, and soy foods. And the overall better life expectancy of the community reflects that fact.

Vegan Doesn't Necessarily Mean Healthy

It's important to understand that one can adopt a vegan or vegetarian diet (perhaps for ethical reasons) and still end up eating very unhealthy foods. Merely avoiding animal foods is not the answer to good health. Remember our first dietary principle: choose whole foods over processed foods. Don't be a junk-food vegan or vegetarian! Yes, studies have shown that vegetarians have a decreased risk of cancer, less obesity, and, depending on the study you look at, possibly greater longevity as well.[21] We would suggest that those studies track not just decreased consumption of unhealthy animal products, but also *an increase in healthy plant-based foods in the diet*—greater consumption of fruits and vegetables, whole grains, and beans and other legumes, with all their corresponding healthy nutrients and micronutrients. In the very large European Prospective Investigation into Cancer and Nutrition (or EPIC) study, four combined lifestyle behaviors were associated with an extra fourteen years of longevity—not smoking, only moderate consumption of alcohol, physical activity, and *the consumption of at least five servings of fruits and vegetables every day.*[22]

Becoming a vegetarian should never be considered a ticket to health all by itself. Doughnuts, French fries, and banana splits are all vegetarian, and not one of them is going to make a top-ten health food list any time soon. A whole foods, plant-based diet stays away from refined grains, highly processed carbohydrates and sugars, and oils. In fact, there have even been studies, like the aforementioned EPIC study, that did not find a significant difference in life expectancy between meat-eaters and vegetarians. But here's a key to interpreting that data: the vegetarians in the EPIC study were eating only half the fiber of the Adventist vegetarians in Loma Linda. That means they were eating far fewer whole plant foods! The Loma Linda vegetarians were eating many more whole foods and plants, and all the healthy fiber and nutrients that they are packaged in. The results speak for themselves—an ordinary population, genetically diverse, with extraordinary health outcomes. As Garth Davis, MD, puts it, "If everyone ate like a Seventh-day Adventist, everyone would have the health of a Seventh-day Adventist."[23]

One person who certainly appears to have the health of a Seventh-day Adventist—or of the rural Chinese he studied—is T. Colin Campbell. Today, in his eighties and still robust and active, he runs a nutritional center, teaches at Cornell, and lectures around the world on the benefits of the whole foods, plant-based diet. Visit his offices in Ithaca, New York, and you can stop for lunch at the famous Moosewood Restaurant across the street—one of the country's original vegetarian outposts. Founded back when not eating animals was considered radical, this venerable establishment has no doubt contributed to Ithaca's reputation as a bastion of unconventional ideas—"ten square miles surrounded by reality," as the locals like to say. "Reality," in America's food landscape, may indeed still be Big Macs, bologna, and bacon cheeseburgers. Meat is still "what's for dinner," more often than not. But thanks to people like Campbell and research like The China Study and the Adventist Health Studies, that reality is shifting. Cultural change can seem slow at times, especially for those who most vividly see a better future, but already the plant-based food movement is strong and growing, and without question it owes a lot to this independent-minded elder statesman.

◡ WHOLE FOODIE TAKEAWAYS ◠

• **Eat mostly plants**—The correlation between diets heavy in animal foods and higher rates of chronic disease has been well established by large epidemiological studies like The China Study and the Adventist Health Studies.

• **Nutritional science needs to be holistic**—Many different forms of research add up to a more comprehensive picture. Approach nutritional science with a skeptical mind and look for patterns, not sensational headlines.

• **The longest-lived population in the world eats a primarily plant-based diet**—If you want to live well into your nineties, eat like an Adventist!

CHAPTER 4

Reverse-Engineering Longevity

Food and Culture in the Blue Zones

"Traditions are not just old-fashioned ways of doing things. They are
tried and true algorithms for keeping people healthy and happy."

—*Michael Pollan*

Do you want to live a long life? At first consideration, there are few who
would say no. But when researchers from the University of Pennsylvania
qualified the question with the addition of various chronic diseases, it soon
became clear that for many, conditions like dementia, incontinence, and lung
failure are a fate worse than death.[1] As the poet E. E. Cummings once wrote,
"Unbeing dead isn't being alive." Human beings want to live long lives, but
they also want to live *healthy* lives—to be vital, able-bodied, and relatively free
of chronic disease. The lure of longevity is certainly less sweet if it only means
extending the pain and suffering of a growing list of physical ailments.

The power of a whole foods, plant-based diet lies in its capacity to
fulfill our twin aspirations to extend our life span *and* our health span. And
perhaps nowhere is this more clearly demonstrated than in the remarkable
work of a journalist and explorer named Dan Buettner, who set out to find
the longest-lived people on earth and learn the secrets of their lifestyles.
His research on these populations, which came to be known as the "Blue
Zones," has offered the world a window into five extraordinary incubators
of human health and vitality. Dotted across the globe, with diverse cultures,
environments, traditions, and genetics, each of these populations has an

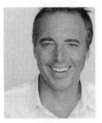

WHOLE FOODIE HERO
Dan Buettner

"The longest-lived people eat a plant-based diet. They eat meat but only as a condiment or a celebration. Nothing they eat has a plastic wrapper."

Contributions: Buettner's Blue Zone research has educated millions about the diet and lifestyle of the world's longest-lived peoples and inspired individuals, communities, cities, and states to adopt Blue Zone principles to "live longer and be happier."

Fun facts: Building on his Blue Zone research, Buettner's latest exploration is a deep dive into the source of human happiness. What is it that makes people happy? Are there common cross-cultural factors that we can discern?

Read this: *The Blue Zones Solution: Eating and Living Like the World's Healthiest People*

Learn more: BlueZones.com

unusual concentration of people who live into their nineties and even beyond one hundred. They have a surprising number of things in common, perhaps the most striking that they all eat a whole foods diet, with, on average, 90% of their calories coming from plant foods.

Buettner's journey into longevity began around the turn of the millennium. For a number of years, he had been leading expeditions around the world, investigating some of history's most mesmerizing mysteries. Why did the Mayan civilization collapse? Did Marco Polo really go to China? What happened to the Anasazi? As a journalist, entrepreneur, Emmy Award–winning producer, traveler, cyclist, holder of multiple Guinness World Records, and go-to *National Geographic* writer, Buettner has lived a life of multiple identities.

Health and diet were hardly front and center in his adventures. He describes himself as once having had a "see food diet"—"I would see food…and eat it."[2] That all changed in 2000, when one particularly captivating mystery drew his attention. The World Health Organization had discovered that Okinawans—residents of the Japanese island made famous by American occupation during World War II—had the longest disability-free life expectancy in the world. Why would one particular island civilization have such an outsize health potential? Buettner had found his next adventure.

With help from the National Institute on Aging and *National Geographic*, he put together a team, flew to Okinawa, and began to investigate local living and eating habits. The more he learned about the lifestyle of this remarkable population of elders, the more convinced he became that he was onto something of real significance. As the project developed, so did its goal. Buettner saw an opportunity, as he puts it, to "reverse-engineer longevity."[3] Research into genetics and longevity, including the well-known Longitudinal Study of Aging Danish Twins, had suggested that genetics account for only 20% to 30% of life span, with the rest due to environmental and lifestyle factors.[4] If *how* we live plays such a large role in *how long* we live, Buettner reasoned, then surely it would be instructive to locate the longest-lived populations and carefully examine their behaviors. He began to look beyond Okinawa for other large concentrations of centenarians, and ask, How do they achieve such remarkable outcomes? Where do they live? What kinds of communities do they have? And perhaps most importantly, what do they eat?

Of course, this is easier said than done. Longevity can be notoriously tricky to determine in older cohorts. Demographers must start in one area with a selection of documented births between ninety and a hundred years earlier and track those people and their lifestyle over almost a century. As Buettner's team closed in on potential populations, they used a blue Sharpie marker to circle the regions on the map—hence the informal name "Blue Zone," which stuck.

Okinawa was the first Blue Zone. Japan as a nation boasts the world's longest life spans, but Okinawans leave their mainland compatriots in the dust. This relatively small tropical island region southwest of mainland Japan has one of the highest ratios of centenarians—6.5 in 10,000 live to be 100. The islanders over sixty-five enjoy the world's highest life expectancy. They have lower rates of disease than Americans in just about every category, with only half the dementia of those of a similar age.

The next Blue Zone that Buettner identified was on the Mediterranean island of Sardinia. If you picture easy-living centenarians taking long naps in hammocks near the turquoise sea, think again—the Blue Zone is specifically an inland region known as Ogliastra, the most mountainous area of the island. The pastoral people of these highlands tend sheep and eke out a simple living amid an unforgiving terrain. It's not exactly an easy life, but it is a long and rewarding one, particularly for men—the longest-lived males on earth are those who tread the rugged paths of Sardinia's mountains.

The third Blue Zone he identified was the Seventh-day Adventist religious group in Loma Linda, California, that you read about in chapter 3. Buettner featured these three Blue Zones in a 2005 *National Geographic* feature that went viral, becoming the third most popular in the esteemed magazine's hundred-year history. A best-selling book followed, but Buettner was not done exploring.

Before long, two more Blue Zones came to light: Ikaria, Greece, and the Nicoya Peninsula of Costa Rica. A relatively remote island not far from the west coast of Turkey, Ikaria has only a little more than eight thousand inhabitants. It has a rugged terrain that contrasts with the warm Mediterranean climate and relaxed lifestyle of its people, who live almost a decade longer than their counterparts in America with half the rates of heart disease.[5] Meanwhile, in Costa Rica's hilly Nicoya region, once used as a refuge by the Contra rebels of neighboring Nicaragua, the *mestizos* (people of combined European and American Indian descent) reach the age of ninety at two and one-half times the rate of northern Americans and have much less cancer, heart disease, and diabetes.[6] This hardy population no longer dies from infectious diseases that once were the scourge of their ancestors, such as dysentery, dengue fever, or malaria; yet, they have also stayed relatively free of the diseases of affluence that afflict Costa Rica's city-dwelling populations.

Buettner and his team spent significant time in each Blue Zone, observing, researching, surveying, and otherwise exploring the lifestyles and daily activities of these remarkable pockets of long-lived peoples. Slowly all five began to yield their secrets, the behaviors most clearly linked to their extraordinary health outcomes. Buettner's plan to reverse-engineer longevity was paying off, as he was able to find critical lifestyle similarities among all the Blue Zones—even though they were spread across the world.

Dietary Secrets of the Centenarians

Among all the lifestyle factors that distinguish the Blue Zones, one of the most significant is diet. Buettner and his team made friends with the local centenarians, watching them in their kitchens and gardens, walking with them in their neighborhoods, and recording their habits as they went about their days. And they asked questions—lots of questions. Buettner acknowledges that it was a complex task: "If you want to know what a one-hundred-year-old ate to live to one hundred, you have to know what they ate their entire life—what they ate as kids, when they were married, when they were middle-aged, when they were sixty, and when they retired. And today you can't just ask them, because they don't remember. So it was a mammoth undertaking."[7]

After years of research, Buettner has reams of carefully constructed demographic data, right alongside the notes and remembrances from his numerous personal journeys to these lands that the Grim Reaper seems reluctant to visit. In addition, with support from Harvard's Walter Willett, he initiated a meta-analysis of every dietary survey done in the last hundred years in each Blue Zone by local and international researchers.

While at first glance the plates of these different peoples might look quite different, a closer look reveals many common patterns. As one example, Buettner points to "Greens and beans. No matter where you go in the Blue

Zones, they are eating a lot of green vegetables and about a cup of beans a day."[8] In one extended study in Ikaria, a cohort was followed for several years, and the researchers found that those who were doing the best at surviving were eating about a half cup of greens and a cup of beans every day.

The types of beans and greens vary, as do the foods that accompany them. In Okinawa they eat soybeans and various green leafy vegetables, together with their favorite food—sweet potatoes—a starchy vegetable that accounted for up to 67% of the islanders' calories in the pre- and postwar periods, when meat was scarce. Rice also plays a key role in the Okinawan diet, and while they love pork, they eat very little by Western standards, generally consuming pork or fish in small quantities just two or three times a week. They eat very few dairy products. Before 1940, 80% of their diet was made up of whole food starches, and they flourished—a fact that may surprise "low-carb" dieters.

The Sardinians love fava beans, chickpeas, fennel, and zucchini. Like many Mediterranean cultures, they eat a generous amount of bread made from both barley and durum wheat, and pasta. They enjoy cheese and milk, almost entirely from goats and sheep. They drink the deep red Cannonau wine from the Grenache grape that thrives on their sun-drenched hillsides. Meat and fish consumption in the Sardinian Blue Zone is generally less than in Mediterranean diets, including those of the coastal dwellers on the same island. (See box, page 84, for further discussion of the Mediterranean diet.)

In the neighboring Mediterranean Blue Zone of Ikaria, the traditional diet includes a variety of wild mountain greens found on the island, along with chickpeas and black-eyed peas. As in Sardinia, the mountain dwellers in Ikaria eat fish less often than those on the coast—in this case due to the legendary rough seas and winds in the area around the island (they are even mentioned in the *Iliad*) that have made fishing a complicated endeavor and limited local supply—and they live longer. Ikarians enjoy pasta and olive oil in accordance with Mediterranean traditions, but they also eat more legumes and potatoes than are typical for other cultures in the region. They eat meat or poultry in small quantities a few times per week, and enjoy a bounty of fresh vegetables, grown locally or in gardens, year-round. They drink coffee and tea and love wine and honey, but eat very little refined sugar or flour. Their reputation for longevity has its roots in antiquity, when the Greeks would visit this island to soak in its hot springs, all the way back in the fifth century BCE, when the island was part of the Athenian Alliance.

The Nicoyans feast on black beans and locally available green vegetables, as part of a diet rich in maize (corn), squash, yams, rice, and tropical fruits. Meat, poultry, dairy products, and fish are common, but limited in terms of overall dietary calories, as well as the occasional egg.[9] Buettner sums it up as follows: "Like residents of other Blue Zones, people here ate a high-carb, moderate-fat, moderate-protein plant-based diet rich in legumes."[10]

The Adventists, as discussed in chapter 3, eat a wide variety of beans, lentils, green vegetables, some nuts, and a variety of other vegetables. Their diets can be mapped on a spectrum from those who eat some meat and/or fish to those who are vegetarian or vegan, but what they all have in common is a focus on real, unprocessed foods. Even those who ate meat did so much less frequently than the average American.

Do you start to see the common patterns emerging? Real, unprocessed foods, mostly plants. Rich in beans and other legumes, whole grains and starchy vegetables, fresh fruits, greens, and other vegetables. In other words, every Blue Zone ate some variation of a whole foods, plant-based diet.

Gardens are common in every one of these regions, often with multiple growing seasons per year, adding to the supply of fresh fruits and vegetables. In fact, most of the food that is consumed in the Blue Zones, Buettner notes, grows within a ten-mile radius of the home.[11] Of course, that's not possible or even desirable for everyone to replicate, but what we can learn from these traditional ways of life, no matter where we live, is to choose whole foods, and include lots of fruits and vegetables.

Another important common factor among the Blue Zone diets that Buettner highlights is their emphasis on carbohydrates, often complex carbohydrates like whole grains, starchy vegetables, and legumes, with much lower levels of animal foods than the Standard American Diet. This flies in the face of the trend toward "low-carb" diets that promote more fats and encourage meat consumption (see chapter 7). Indeed, when it comes to meat and other animal foods, the evidence from the Blue Zones clearly suggests that a significant reduction is in order. The meta-analysis of Blue Zone diets that Buettner and his team conducted revealed that on average, over the entire long lifetimes of the elders, the Blue Zone diets were 90% plant-based, 10% animal products.

Among these longest-lived people, only a small percentage of the Adventists cut out animal foods completely. Every other Blue Zone diet includes meat or fish of various kinds, but in very limited amounts. The longest-lived women in the world, in Okinawa, ate a little fish and pork.

The Mediterranean Diet: More than Olive Oil and Red Wine

With two of the world's five Blue Zones located in the Mediterranean, clearly there is a connection between longevity and the traditional eating habits of those who live on the shores of Homer's "wine-dark sea." Some have suggested as much, pointing out that the populations of Crete, Greece, and Southern Italy seem to have better health outcomes, at least in recent history, even as they have worse medical care.

So what is the Mediterranean diet? It's largely based around vegetables, fruits, grains, legumes, fish, and eggs, along with some meat, dairy, olive oil, and red wine. Which of those foods do you think Americans have come to primarily associate with the Mediterranean diet? Vegetables, whole grains, and beans? Sadly, no. To most people it seems to be synonymous with "olive oil and red wine"! Too many who claim to eat this diet simply *add* olive oil and red wine to what they were already eating, as if they were miracle health foods.

There is little evidence that this is true. Olive oil is one of the most calorie-dense foods that exists (four thousand calories per pound),

The longest-lived men in the world, in Sardinia, ate pork, goat, and lamb, but traditionally only on special occasions. And perhaps the overall longest-lived people in the entire world that we know of are the "vegetarians" of Loma Linda, eating mostly fruits, vegetables, unprocessed starch foods, beans, and nuts, with small amounts of animal products added by some as well.

It is also worth noting that the Blue Zones consume very little milk or milk products, and when they do it tends to come from sheep and goats. Cow's milk and cheese are almost entirely absent, with the exception of the vegetarians and meat-eaters among the Loma Linda Adventists.

Another notable feature of the Blue Zones diets is not what they eat, but what they drink. Most Blue Zones keep it simple—water, coffee, tea, and a little wine. They rarely drink fruit juices, and completely avoid the sodas,

and has lost all the healthy fiber and nearly all the nutrients of the olive in the extraction process. Nor is olive oil consumption the best or most efficient means of getting the healthy polyphenols and plant sterols that advocates point to in their health claims. All in all, there is scant evidence for health sanctification, and plenty of reason for caution.

As far as red wine goes, we can appreciate the importance it plays in the Mediterranean lifestyle. Health is never a story only about food, and wine may play a role in bringing people together, amplifying our convivial and relational nature. None of that, of course, means that wine should be considered a health food or consumed in excess. Indeed, there is significant evidence to link alcohol consumption and certain cancers[16]—all the more reason to practice moderation if you choose to consume it at all.

It is likely that the real nutritional engine of the Mediterranean diet was always the higher amount of fruits, vegetables, whole grains, and legumes, and the fact that when animal foods were consumed, it was in relatively modest amounts. The Mediterranean Blue Zones, with their even lower proportion of animal foods and high levels of fruit and vegetable consumption, support this conclusion.

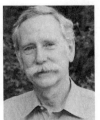

WHOLE FOODIE HERO
Walter C. Willett, MD

"A diet rich in fruits and vegetables plays a role in reducing the risk of all major causes of illness and death."

Contributions: As chair of the Harvard School of Public Health's Department of Nutrition, Willett has been a giant in the field, and a leading voice in the efforts to ameliorate America's chronic disease epidemic. He assisted Dan Buettner with the Blue Zones dietary meta-analysis, and is the most widely cited academic in the field of nutrition.

Fun facts: The *Boston Globe* once described Willett as "the world's most influential nutritionist."

Read this: *Eat, Drink, and Be Healthy: The Harvard Medical School Guide to Healthy Eating*

Learn more: hsph.harvard.edu/nutritionsource

sports drinks, energy drinks, sugary cocktails, Frappuccinos, and other calorie-laden beverages common in the United States. Adventists recommend seven glasses of water a day, and are the only Blue Zone population that abstains from alcohol. Okinawans tend to have a glass of tea near them constantly, often green tea, which has been shown to have all kinds of health benefits. Ikarians, Sardinians, and Nicoyans all love to drink coffee.

Nudges and Defaults

It is important to remember that the elders of the Blue Zones were not consciously trying to be fit, healthy, slim, or long lived. They were not deliberately following a "longevity diet" or restricting certain foods because they perceived them as "bad." "Longevity happened to these people," Buettner explains. "They didn't seek it out."[12] They were certainly not reading the latest nutritional science and trying to apply it in their kitchens, gardens, and dining rooms. In these often-remote regions of the world, whole healthy plant foods were simply the cheapest and easiest to get. These people valued convenience in their lives as much as we do, and their unusual health outcomes are largely due to lifestyles that were traditional and easy to maintain. From walking to gardening to eating to cooking to socializing to living with a strong sense of faith and purpose, they followed the patterns that fit conveniently into their community and culture. Their way of life, from dawn to dusk, just happened to also support healthy, positive, life-enhancing behaviors. And they lived in tight-knit social networks that consistently reinforced the same.

While many aspects of the Blue Zones lifestyle harken back to a simpler time and a more traditional diet, it would be a mistake to think that the answer to our modern dietary dilemmas is just to return to the good old days and live like our ancestors. The Blue Zones represent a rare combination of cultural, geographical, and historical conditions. They were lucky enough to benefit from the medical breakthroughs of modernity, but remote enough to escape its nutritional downsides. On the one hand, each of these regions was close enough to the developed world to benefit from public health policy and its ability to end the scourge of infectious disease. No longer were people dying young of dysentery or malaria. On the other hand, they were just far enough removed from the faster-changing urban areas to avoid being overrun by Western eating habits and the new modern epidemics of chronic disease. These geographic sweet spots fortuitously fell between the cracks of cultural trends that overlapped in most parts of the world. And the rare convergence of conditions that made them possible is already past.

There are unlikely to be more Blue Zones discovered, Buettner says, although he continues to search. And the existing five are already under pressure—from globalization, development, Western eating habits, and the "diseases of affluence" that come with them. In Okinawa, people under sixty now have *higher* rates of chronic disease than Americans! As modernity encroaches, so does the modern lifestyle with its industrial food systems, its greater wealth, and its rise in processed food, meat, and dairy consumption. In his trips Buettner has noticed the changes. "If you're invited to dinner by a Sardinian today, it's like they are barbecuing a petting zoo," he says, with a pained laugh. "They'll start with prosciutto, and then lamb, and then pork. It's the complete opposite of the diet that helped make them a Blue Zone."[13]

Soon, as the longest lives on earth come to an end, the Blue Zones will be gone, with the possible exception of Loma Linda, a community that is more intentional in preserving its lifestyle. But thanks to Buettner and his team, their secrets are with us forever—impeccably researched, clearly elucidated, and highly replicable. We can apply their longevity principles, today, no matter where in the world we live. The Adventists are prime examples of this. Their Blue Zone wasn't built on ancient traditions or carefully protected by a quirk of geography. Their religious faith gave them strong-enough conviction and a rich and supportive social network with which to build a barrier against the unhealthy habits of the modern world. We may not be inclined to adopt their faith, but we can learn something from their lifestyle. "To make it to age one hundred, you have to have won the genetic lottery," Buettner concedes. "But most of us have the capacity to make it well into our early nineties and largely without chronic disease. As the Adventists demonstrate, the average person's life expectancy could increase by ten to twelve years by adopting a Blue Zones lifestyle."[14]

Buettner has spent much of the last decade developing methods to bring the longevity secrets to municipalities and even states across America. He has worked intensely to research and develop best practices for embedding Blue Zone principles in places that are rife with obesity, chronic disease, and the food and lifestyle options that create them. Since 2009, Blue Zones Projects are now active in thirty-one American cities. Their approach is light on the rhetoric, focused on education, and all about working with communities— leaders, healthcare organizations, politicians, civic organizations, business leaders, school leaders, students—to get real buy-in.

The key lesson from the Blue Zones that underlies these efforts is this: deep and lasting change happens through what Buettner calls "nudges and defaults" rather than organized, top-down intervention. What the Blue Zones show us is that there are a thousand small ways in which our lives can be set up to *nudge* us in the direction of healthy decisions. They also show that convenience matters—we need to ensure that our *defaults* become the healthy options, not the disease-promoting ones.

We all know how difficult it can be to change habits, eating or otherwise, through personal willpower alone. In part this is because our individual habits are intricately connected to every other thing about ourselves and our lives. Diets, in particular, don't work in isolation. If we don't live in an environment that supports those changes, or connect with a social network that embodies and encourages them, they will be much more difficult to sustain. However, the Blue Zones demonstrate the powerful flip side of this truth: when we do live in the right environment and community, healthy living can become the norm.

With this in mind, Buettner and his team focus on improving the options on the menu in local restaurants, increasing access to community gardens, installing new walking and biking paths, encouraging grocery stores to put healthy foods right near the checkouts, enrolling local schools in Blue Zone projects, making it possible for more kids to walk to school, setting up social support networks for friends and families, banning smoking in public places, encouraging volunteering and other purposeful activities, and setting up workshops, social events, potlucks, and so on. All of these changes create what Buettner calls "a healthy swarm of nudges and defaults"[15] that inspire better eating and better living.

The results have been remarkable, to say the least. In one project, the Blue Zones team worked in three southern California cities—Manhattan Beach, Hermosa Beach, and Redondo Beach (known as the Beach Cities)—and teamed with Gallup to measure the progress. After three years they saw a 14% drop in obesity levels, which represented a savings of more than $2.3 million a year in health costs. They saw a 28% drop in the smoking rate, which represented another $6.97 million savings in health costs. 10% more residents were exercising regularly, and rates of both diabetes and high blood pressure were down. Childhood obesity has fallen an impressive 50%. Other cities have shown similarly striking changes.

Read between the lines of these initiatives and you see another theme: a reinvigoration of America's civic architecture. Social scientists have worried for years about the breakdown of America's rich civic society. The Blue Zone Project is a means of appealing directly to our sense of civic pride and engagement, and of encouraging people and communities to work together to improve our health outcomes. If you're inspired by the stories you've read in this chapter, look no further than your own community for ways to promote health and longevity. Can you team up with like-minded friends to create a healthy-eating support network? What are your kids eating at school, and could you help to improve it? Can you join or start a community garden? Is there a local nonprofit where you could volunteer? The possibilities for creating healthy nudges and defaults are endless.

⌒ WHOLE FOODIE TAKEAWAYS ⌒

• **Live longer, better!**—The longest-lived populations in the world, with extraordinarily low rates of chronic disease, each eat a variation on a whole foods, predominantly plant-based diet.
• **Create healthy nudges and defaults**—If you want to change your habits, you need to set up your environment so the healthy option becomes the default option.

CHAPTER 5

Let Food Be Thy Medicine

Using Diet to Prevent and Reverse Heart Disease

"When diet is wrong, medicine is of no use.
When diet is correct, medicine is of no need."

—*Ayurvedic proverb*

Still groggy from being sedated, Paul Chatlin lay on a gurney contemplating the worst news of his life. After months of chest pain, he had just undergone a diagnostic heart catheterization, and it showed a right artery that was 100% blocked, two others at 65%, leaky valves, an enlarged heart, and a heart murmur to boot. The doctors said he needed a heart bypass, and fast. The only question was, would it be a triple or a quadruple? At just fifty-six, his life was in immediate danger.

Unfortunately, Chatlin's predicament is anything but rare in America today, where more than three hundred thousand people get heart bypass surgery every year, often in their fifties and sixties. Many won't live out the next decade. And even for those for whom heart disease is not a death sentence, it is often a life sentence, a harbinger of physical decline and increasing debilitation. Killing more than 375,000 Americans a year, heart disease remains the number-one cause of death in the United States. It is also the leading cause of death worldwide, taking more than 17.3 million lives annually.[1] Sadly, precious few among those millions are ever given the choice that Chatlin's doctor gave him, just minutes before he was wheeled into the operating room: "Would you consider plant-based nutrition as an alternative to bypass surgery?"

Chatlin, a telecommunications consultant from the Detroit suburbs, had no idea what "plant-based nutrition" meant, but he knew that anything was preferable to a heart bypass. His own father and several other men in his family had never been quite the same after their surgeries. He looked up at his doctor and said, "Yes."

Chatlin didn't know it, but he had won the lottery that day. He was already lucky, thanks to a family connection, to be a patient at the world-famous Cleveland Clinic—one of the top facilities in the world for the treatment of heart disease. Even more remarkably, out of the hundreds of doctors he could have been assigned to, he had ended up with one of only a handful who were familiar with, and who advocated, plant-based nutrition. As Chatlin lay on his gurney, his doctor got out his phone and dialed his mentor, Caldwell Esselstyn, MD, and despite the late hour, "Essy" took the call.

Dr. Esselstyn's message to Chatlin that night was short and sweet: "Go home. I'll give you a call tomorrow morning." He did just that, at eight a.m., outlining his unconventional approach to heart disease: a plant-based nutritional program that treats both the symptoms *and* the underlying disease itself. Chatlin listened carefully. Chance may have opened a previously unseen door, but now it was up to him to walk through it. And the first step, he recalls, was "taking 95% of the food in my kitchen and donating it to charity."[2] Then he went shopping—in the produce section.

For those accustomed to a Standard American Diet, switching to plant-based nutrition involves a radical remaking of what's on the plate and in the pantry. It means changing a lifetime of habits, learning new skills, and developing new tastes. As we'll discuss in chapter 12, some people do best with a slow, step-by-step transition, while others choose to go all in, all at once. Chatlin belonged to the latter group, at least in part due to the severity of his disease. He changed his diet, immediately and completely. And his health changed just as fast. Within three weeks his angina (chest pain) disappeared. Over the next year his cholesterol level dropped from 309 to 122, he shed more than forty pounds, and his energy levels improved significantly.

Heart Disease 101

Heart disease, or coronary heart disease, is an umbrella term for a number of distinct but often-related conditions, including high blood pressure or hypertension, heart attack, stroke, and heart failure.

Many of these conditions stem from a hardening and/or narrowing of the arteries and their endothelial cells (arteriosclerosis or atherosclerosis), caused by a buildup on the artery walls of plaques, which are made up of fats, cholesterol, and other substances.

When these plaques rupture or burst, they can trigger a blood clot, blocking the artery and causing a heart attack or stroke. The narrowing of the arteries also contributes to an increase in blood pressure.

While there is still much being learned about the exact mechanisms of heart disease, most experts agree that elevated cholesterol (including the "bad" LDL cholesterol) is a critical risk factor.

As you might imagine, with a story like this to tell, you would be hard-pressed to find a more passionate evangelist for the benefits of a whole foods, plant-based diet than Chatlin. But his tale is hardly unique— particularly not among patients of Dr. Esselstyn.

Clinical Pioneers of Plant-Based Nutrition

Caldwell Esselstyn did not train as a cardiologist. In the late 1960s, however, an accident of alphabetical proximity meant that this thyroid surgeon shared a locker at the Cleveland Clinic with René Favaloro, the celebrated Argentinian cardiac surgeon who performed the first heart bypass surgery in 1967. Esselstyn and Favaloro talked at length about the causes and consequences of heart disease. Favaloro's innovative approach to surgery would go on to affect tens of thousands of lives over the next decades, but did little to address the underlying issues that put people on the operating table in the first place. Esselstyn, on the other hand, grew increasingly disillusioned with the conventional approach to "America's silent killer."

Heart disease, like other common American diseases, including breast cancer, prostate cancer, colon cancer, and diabetes, has been found to be rare in parts of the world that eat more traditional diets. But once those same regions adopted more Western-style diets, with higher levels of animal products and processed food, disease rates skyrocketed. This was true not just in China but in Japan and in parts of Africa. Researchers also noted that when individuals moved to regions of the world where these diseases were prevalent, they would soon develop the same problems as the communities around them. This tells us that the problem is not genetics, as many believed. Genetics may load the gun, as they say, but diet pulls the trigger.

Research also shows that heart disease is not just a problem of the elderly. Autopsies of fallen soldiers in Vietnam and Korea revealed that heart disease was common even in the young—80% of the young American troops showed signs of it in their arteries. (It was largely absent in the Asian soldiers.)[3] Studies have shown that by the age of ten, nearly all children show fatty streaks on the arteries, the first signs of arterial damage, and that these may even begin developing in the womb.[4] Heart disease does not just appear right before a heart attack. Most Americans already have it. As Esselstyn reviewed all this research, he began to wonder. Could heart disease be stopped? And could it be done through diet?

He was not the first to ask these questions. In the late 1950s, a young man named Nathan Pritikin had been diagnosed with heart disease at just forty-two years of age. Through a long experimentation with diet, he eventually reversed his disease. In 1975, he opened up a "longevity center" in California to share his regimen, which was essentially a whole foods, primarily plant-based diet, along with exercise every day. Pritikin's patients got better—a lot better! Risk factors for heart disease improved across the board, cholesterol went down, and arterial function and blood flow improved, along with a host of other health transformations. Pritikin's work attracted a great

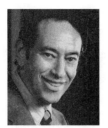

WHOLE FOODIE HERO
Nathan Pritikin

"All I'm trying to do is wipe out heart disease, diabetes, hypertension, and obesity."

Contributions: Pritikin was one of the very first to show that a whole foods, plant-based diet could significantly affect chronic disease. After reversing his own disease through diet, he founded the Pritikin Longevity Center where his regimen produced impressive results in reversing many chronic conditions.

Fun facts: Pritikin was a prolific inventor who held patents in chemistry, physics, and electronics.

Learn more: pritikin.com

deal of attention in his day, but without medical credentials or controlled trials, he was never fully accepted by the establishment. Since his death, more than 100 studies in peer-reviewed journals have validated the program's effectiveness. Meanwhile, however, the task of scientifically demonstrating that diet and lifestyle change could reverse heart disease was being taken up by an independent-minded young physician from the Lone Star State.

Dean Ornish, MD, had been curious about how diet and lifestyle—a whole foods, plant-based diet, moderate exercise, yoga and meditation, and social support (love and intimacy)—might impact heart disease since his medical school days. In fact, he conducted his first small study in 1977 after his second year at Baylor College of Medicine in Houston, asking Dr. Antonio Gotto, the chief of medicine there, to refer heart patients to him so he could conduct an experiment to see whether yoga and a vegetarian diet could reverse heart disease. This was long before the days when there was a yoga studio on every other block—such ideas were part of the just-emerging counterculture. His skeptical supervisor asked, "Should I say I'm referring patients to a swami?" but Ornish won him over by calling it "stress management training and dietary changes" and got ten participants enrolled.[5] This was the heyday of bypass surgery, so the only patients who were referred to him were those who were too sick to undergo surgery or had refused it.

Eight of the ten participants showed significant improvement in blood flow to the heart after only one month. This was the first study showing that heart disease could be reversed by lifestyle changes alone.[6]

Ornish completed medical school in 1980 and began a new study—this time, a randomized controlled trial of forty-eight patients. After only twenty-four days, the patients who made comprehensive lifestyle changes showed improvement (reversal) in their heart disease, whereas those in the randomized control group got worse. This, the first randomized controlled trial showing that lifestyle changes alone could reverse heart disease, was published in the *Journal of the American Medical Association.*

The results of these two studies were both statistically significant and clinically significant, and Ornish published his first best-selling book on the topic in 1982.

After completing his medical training at Harvard Medical School and Massachusetts General Hospital, he moved to Sausalito, California, became a clinical professor of medicine at UCSF, and established the nonprofit Preventive Medicine Institute to continue the research. In 1984, he launched the Lifestyle Heart Trial.

Back in Cleveland, Esselstyn was also developing a study. He had encountered some resistance from the establishment. Most senior cardiologists at the Cleveland Clinic, he writes, "did not believe there was a connection between diet and coronary disease."[7] Nevertheless, in 1985, the Department of Cardiology agreed to participate in his first proposed study. It would refer patients to him—primarily those for whom bypass surgery or angioplasty had failed, and several who had been told there was nothing more that could be done for them. Esselstyn's hypothesis was that plant-based nutrition could reduce their cholesterol levels to below 150 mg/dL (closer to the level seen in those traditional cultures that had no heart disease) and in so doing, slow or halt the disease process. By 1988 a cohort of twenty-four people with severe, progressive coronary artery disease was eating a very

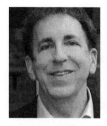

WHOLE FOODIE HERO
Dean Ornish, MD

"I don't understand why asking people to eat a well-balanced vegetarian diet is considered drastic, while it is medically conservative to cut people open."

Contributions: Dr. Ornish's research proved for the first time that heart disease could be prevented and reversed through diet and lifestyle changes.

Fun facts: The stress-management techniques used in Dr. Ornish's Lifestyle Heart Trial were partially inspired by his friend and teacher Swami Satchidananda, the Indian spiritual leader who built the ecumenical LOTUS temple.

Read this: *The Spectrum: A Scientifically Proven Program to Feel Better, Live Longer, Lose Weight, and Gain Health*

Learn more: ornish.com

low-fat, plant-based diet under his supervision.

From a dietary standpoint, Ornish's and Esselstyn's studies were very similar. However, unlike Esselstyn, who instructed patients to continue their medications, Ornish did not use cholesterol-lowering medications in his study. Moreover, he stipulated other lifestyle changes in addition to the nutritional component, including relaxation techniques (yoga and meditation), moderate exercise, smoking cessation, and participation in a support group—interventions he believes are also critical to the success of the program. His study included forty-eight patients who were randomized into two groups: twenty-eight of the patients made the recommended diet and lifestyle changes, while the other twenty served as a control group, following standard medical treatment and dietary advice from the American Heart Association.

Ornish's work was the first to be made public. In 1990 he published the one-year results. Most of the experimental group reported *a complete or nearly complete disappearance of chest pains.* But patients not only *felt* better, they *were* better. When measurements were taken of their narrowed arteries using angiograms (a form of arterial X-ray), 82% showed an increased diameter (reversal). Only one patient who had poor adherence showed significant progression (worsening).

The implications of these data were revolutionary: coronary artery disease not only could be halted through lifestyle change, it could be *reversed*. This group also showed a 37.2% reduction in LDL or "bad" cholesterol. In contrast, patients in the usual-care control group, who made more moderate changes in lifestyle, reduced LDL cholesterol levels by only 6%, had a 165.5% *increase* in reported frequency of chest pains, and showed *progression* (worsening) in narrowing of the coronary arteries.[8]

Five-year results from the study continued to turn conventional wisdom about heart disease on its head. The experimental group showed further improvements in arterial blockages (an average of 8% improvement) and experienced 2.5 times fewer cardiac events than the control group, whose measurements worsened by 28%. There was a dose-response correlation between adherence to Ornish's lifestyle program and changes in their coronary arteries—at any age. Also, there was a *400% increase in blood flow to the heart* in the experimental group patients when compared to the randomized control group as measured by cardiac PET scans. These results were published in the *Lancet* and the *Journal of the American Medical Association*, two of the most prestigious medical journals in the world.[9]

Meanwhile, Esselstyn was getting similarly impressive results from his own study. After five years, average cholesterol levels among those who adhered to the program were almost halved. Among those patients on whom he was able to conduct follow-up angiograms, none showed further narrowing of the arteries, and approximately 70% showed evidence of reversal. Most significantly, no new cardiac disorders or other evidence of heart disease progression occurred during the twelve years of the study, compared with forty-nine incidents among those same patients prior to the study. Among patients who dropped out of the program and returned to their regular diet,

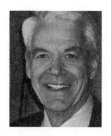

WHOLE FOODIE HERO
Caldwell B. Esselstyn Jr., MD

"Coronary artery disease is a benign food-borne illness which need never exist or progress."

Contributions: The Esselstyn Heart Trial scientifically demonstrates the power of a whole foods, plant-based diet in reversing heart disease.

Fun facts: Esselstyn competed in the 1956 Melbourne Olympics as a part of the Yale crew team. The crew came home with the gold medal.

Read this: *Prevent and Reverse Heart Disease: The Revolutionary, Scientifically Proven, Nutrition-Based Cure*

Learn more: dresselstyn.com

there were thirteen new cardiac incidents, including one death.[10]

In 2006, Esselstyn launched a second, larger study, this time following 198 patients who adopted his plant-based nutritional program. In 2014 he published the results: of those who complied with the diet, 93% experienced improvement in angina symptoms. And only one patient experienced a major cardiovascular event due to recurrent disease (a stroke)—demonstrating that his diet was protective for 99.4% of patients who followed it. In comparison, among the twenty-one participants who did not adhere to the program, thirteen experienced further cardiac events, including two deaths.[11]

Ornish's and Esselstyn's studies represent a dramatic medical breakthrough. Until that point the best that drugs and surgical treatments could do was *manage* heart disease. They ended up doing something few even believed was possible: they showed that heart disease is *reversible.* And they did it with lifestyle interventions that had no negative side effects. Simply by stopping eating foods that were clogging up their arteries and instead eating healthy plant-based fare (and in Ornish's program, practicing relaxation techniques, exercising, and participating in a support group), their patients began to heal—at any age. Their remarkable turnarounds show that it's never too late when it comes to heart disease.

It's hard to overstate how significant this research is. It takes the suggested correlations of observational science such as The China Study or the Adventist Health Studies and puts them to the test in controlled clinical settings, showing the extraordinary power of whole plant foods to succeed where the best of modern medicine has fallen short. So how were these groundbreaking results received by the nutritional establishment and the general public? Initially, Ornish recalls, "We had a lot of opposition to our work because it didn't fit within the conventional paradigm."[12] But without question, the last decades have seen a massive uptick in our culture's general appreciation of the role of diet in heart disease. Ornish has become a hero to many and something of a health celebrity, thanks in part to some high-profile patients like Bill Clinton. In 2010, Medicare agreed to offer coverage for Ornish's program and most insurance companies now do so as well. Others, like Esselstyn, have confirmed the viability of this approach and added their own significant evidence to the mix.

Recently the American College of Cardiology had its first plant-based president, Dr. Kim Williams, who remarked upon assuming the position: "Wouldn't it be a laudable goal…to put ourselves out of business within a generation or two?"[13] Williams chaired a six-hour symposium on lifestyle medicine, the first ever at the ACC, at its most recent annual scientific session in Chicago, with Ornish as a speaker, and several hundred cardiologists attended, with many more being turned away at the door.

However, people like Williams are still the exception, not the rule. When it comes to the overall medical establishment, remarkably little has changed. It's almost as if someone found a cure for our number-one killer, and no one noticed or cared. Far too many people still don't seem to have gotten the memo, and unfortunately this includes many doctors. The majority of medical professionals and institutions still operate as if we do not have evidence that a whole foods, plant-based diet can prevent and reverse heart disease—the cause of hundreds of thousands of deaths and billions of dollars in healthcare costs annually, not to mention untold suffering across the nation and globe. And culture in general seems to view heart disease as if it were a natural and even inevitable consequence of old age, rather than a preventable foodborne illness.

Yet Ornish is hopeful that a shift is beginning. "There has been a convergence of forces that I think are finally making this the right idea at the right time," he says. "The limitations and costs of conventional drugs and surgery are becoming increasingly clear, the power of lifestyle change is also much more well-documented, preventative measures are becoming increasingly incentivized in today's healthcare system, and Medicare and most of the commercial insurance companies are making it more financially sustainable and attractive for physicians and other healthcare professionals to offer our lifestyle medicine program."[14]

We hope that the next decade proves Ornish's optimism to be well founded. As Dr. Greger puts it, "The fact is, there's only one diet ever that has been proven to reverse the number-one killer of men and women in this country—a whole foods, plant-based diet. So shouldn't that be the default recommended diet until proven otherwise? Even if that's all it could do— reverse heart disease—the whole debate should be over!"[15]

And yet, amazingly, that's not all it can do. Ornish has recently had promising results using his program in a randomized controlled trial with early-stage prostate cancer patients and hopes to undertake a similar trial with early-stage breast cancer patients. A whole foods, plant-based diet has been shown to significantly affect a whole host of other chronic conditions, including type 2 diabetes (see chapter 6), colon cancer, Alzheimer's disease, high cholesterol, high blood pressure, and Parkinson's disease.

The Big (Saturated) Fat Debate

It's impossible to raise the issue of a nutritional answer to heart disease without running headlong into the debate over dietary fat and its

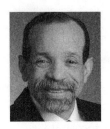

WHOLE FOODIE HERO
Kim Williams, MD

"I personally have had good friends pass away from things that diet could have cured. Only a few of my colleagues have agreed to take a critical look at the data on diet. After they do, they always move toward plant-based nutrition."

Contributions: As president of the American College of Cardiology, Dr. Williams used his prominent position to advocate for the cardiovascular benefits of a plant-based diet.

Fun facts: In 2003, despite eating what he had thought was a healthy diet, Williams was diagnosed with high cholesterol. After he switched to an entirely plant-based diet, his blood cholesterol dropped dramatically.

relationship to cholesterol. As you know from chapter 1, we don't love the idea of focusing on individual nutrients like saturated fat instead of whole foods, given that we don't eat nutrients, we eat food. However, for the sake of helping you navigate nutritional concepts that you'll inevitably be confronted with, let's take a moment to talk about saturated fat.

Official American dietary guidelines encourage us to reduce our consumption of this particular type of fat because of long-established links to heart disease. What that means, in practice, is reducing consumption of animal products, like red meat, chicken, fish, eggs, butter, and milk, since saturated fat is rarely found in significant amounts in plants (coconut oil and palm oil being notable exceptions).

Consumption of saturated fat has been shown to raise LDL (or "bad") cholesterol, which represents a significant risk factor for clogging the arteries. Other foods that raise LDL cholesterol include trans fats (a type of processed unsaturated fat found in animal products and hydrogenated vegetable oils) and dietary cholesterol (cholesterol we consume when we eat animal foods). A whole foods, plant-based diet reduces each of those three to minimal levels, which goes a long way toward explaining its success in treating heart disease.

The connections between saturated fat, cholesterol, and heart disease were first made in the late '70s and early '80s, the discovery being largely driven by the work of American scientist Ancel Keys, who noticed a strong correlation between populations that consumed a lot of saturated fat and high rates of heart disease. His research, and others', led to the framing of saturated fat as deeply implicated in heart disease. This categorization was not undeserved, but people fell into the common trap of blaming everything on a scapegoat nutrient rather than on actual foods. Over time, saturated fat was reduced in the public mind to just "fat," and an obsession with "low-fat" foods followed.

Unfortunately, nutrition is inevitably more complex than that. Fat in itself is not good or bad for you—but certain foods are good or bad for you. High saturated fat content is a likely marker for a poor diet, high in animal foods and highly processed foods.

Some years after Keys' work was published, studies began to question whether saturated fat was the singular evil it had been made out to be. Sure enough, they found that other factors were implicated in heart disease as well. Some fingered refined sugars and highly processed foods. Others pointed to animal protein. But too quickly the reasonable message that "saturated fat isn't our only problem" became the dangerous message that "saturated fat isn't a problem at all," which, on the cover of *Time* magazine, got translated into the 2014 headline "Eat Butter!"

Over the last few years, you may well have encountered such articles, declaring that saturated fat has been exonerated, or that its link to heart disease is unproven, and therefore we should just go back to enthusiastically enjoying meat, butter, and other high-saturated-fat foods without concern. Popular authors Nina Teicholz and Gary Taubes have been among the most outspoken promoters of this point of view, along with celebrity doctor Mark Hyman.

These conclusions are based on a few highly criticized and problematic studies, and the overall science does not back them up.[16] Yale's David Katz

Fixing Your Numbers Is Not Enough

When you go to your doctor and are told that your cholesterol is elevated, or that your blood pressure is too high, you're likely to be prescribed medications to bring those numbers down. It's important to understand that those numbers are *indicators* of the disease, not the disease itself. The medications will adjust the indicators, rather than addressing the underlying causes of the problems. This is a common practice in modern medicine. Many doctors and drug companies speak about high cholesterol as if it's a disease in and of itself, when in fact, it is not. The disease is damaged arteries; high cholesterol is just a warning sign. Statins will improve your cholesterol numbers, but they will do little to reverse cardiovascular disease in your arteries.

Imagine that you have a leaky pipe in your roof. You can't see the pipe, but one day you notice a water mark on the ceiling— an ugly stain spreading across your paintwork. That mark is not your real problem—the leaky pipe is. If all you do is repaint the ceiling, you don't fix the problem, you just remove the evidence. You may even forget, for a while, that there's anything wrong, until you wake up one morning to a flooded living room. In the same way, "improving your numbers" through medication alone can lead to a false sense of security about the underlying condition. People continue the bad habits that damage their hearts and wreak havoc on their health, while thinking they are doing better.

This is not to say cholesterol numbers don't matter, or that cholesterol-lowering drugs cannot be useful, even lifesaving, in certain circumstances. But there's a big difference between *earning* good biometrics through lifestyle change and *manipulating* your biometrics with medication. If you want to unclog your arteries—not merely paint over the evidence of their disease—eating a whole foods, plant-based diet is the way to achieve that goal, sustainably. Then your low numbers will be a true indicator of the health you've gained.

clarifies the issue, writing, "We do, indeed, have evidence that saturated fat is not, and never was, our lone dietary peril. Excesses of calories, sugar, refined starch, sodium, and transfats—among others—share in that indictment."[17] However, he strongly criticizes people who "take just such evidence and pretend it suddenly means lard is manna from heaven."[18] He goes on to point out that all of the world's best diets, associated with the best health outcomes, including the Blue Zone diets, are notably low in saturated fat, due to minimal animal foods. In other words, you don't need to worry about saturated fat *if* you simply eat whole foods, mostly plants.

Currently the best scientific evidence we have tells us that meat, eggs, cheese, dairy, and yes, the saturated fats and animal proteins that go along with them should be minimized in a healthy diet—along with highly processed food and added sugars. Our recommendation is to limit animal products to 10% or less of your calories. Those who already have advanced heart disease or certain other conditions may want to more significantly cut back on animal products, in line with Ornish's and Esselstyn's recommendations. Ignore the noise; focus on whole foods, follow the sober science, and you'll enjoy a healthy heart for a long time. Oh, and Ancel Keys, promoter of a Mediterranean-style diet rich in fruits and vegetables, may have had the last laugh. He retired to his Italian home, near the Mediterranean Sea—and lived just two months shy of his 101st birthday.

A Rising Tide

We are hopeful that in the not-too-distant future there will come a day when someone like Paul Chatlin does not have to win the lottery to hear about the benefits of a whole foods, plant-based diet and be offered it as an alternative to surgery. The medical establishment is changing gradually, doctor by doctor. But as Ornish reminds us, the establishment is never where real change begins.

Among those working hardest today to raise awareness of the healing power of a whole foods, plant-based diet and help people stick to it is Chatlin himself. As his own health began to turn around, he made a promise: he was going to do something to give others the opportunity he'd been given. "When I first started my journey, I called a hundred and fifty doctors' offices to let them know about the power of plant-based nutrition," he recalls. "I got one call back."[19] Finally, in 2014, he found an integrative cardiologist, Joel Kahn, MD.

Kahn, who practices in Detroit, had been eating a plant-based diet himself since the late '70s, but it was only when he stumbled upon Ornish's research in *The Lancet*, just after he completed his advanced cardiology fellowship, that he made the connection between the food on his plate and the patients he saw every day. "At first I thought it was nonsense!" he remembers. "I'd just spent seven years learning to treat heart disease with balloons inserted into arteries, and here's this guy I've never heard of saying he can do it with diet."[20] But he was intrigued. He read the article twenty-five times, and then started telling all his patients to read it.

Chatlin invited Kahn to partner with him in forming a support group for heart disease patients who wanted to make the transition. They scheduled their first meeting for a cold February evening at the hospital where Kahn worked. "The room was designed to hold sixty people," he recalls, "but we ended up with more than double that number packed in. To this day, I have no idea where they all came from."[21] The next month, 150 people showed up. The medical establishment may not have been open to Chatlin's message, but patients were. And they told their friends and loved ones about it.

Today, the Plant-Based Nutrition Support Group (PBNSG) has close to three thousand members—men and women, young and old, who are using a whole foods, plant-based diet to lose weight, reverse heart disease or diabetes, control hypertension, get off medications, and much more. "We started out as a cardiac support group," Chatlin recalls, "but then I realized it was selfish of me to think that that's all it should be, so I expanded it."[22]

Monthly meetings, featuring talks by luminaries in the field, are often attended by several hundred to a thousand members. In addition PBNSG offers small-group local meetings, nutritional tours of grocery stores, and community walks. It works with local restaurants to get more plant-based options on menus, and is developing a plant-based nutrition curriculum to be taught in medical schools. "I realized there wasn't much hope for change with established physicians. I decided to focus on *future* doctors,"[23] Chatlin says. Medical students from five Detroit metro-area colleges can now get credit for attending PBNSG lectures, and Chatlin makes sure every one of his distinguished guests, who have included T. Colin Campbell, Caldwell Esselstyn, Joel Fuhrman, John McDougall, and many more, speaks at a local medical school as part of his or her visit.

In a medical world that does not yet embrace the power of plant-based nutrition to heal and cure the chronic diseases of our sick nation, PBNSG meetings provide encouragement and camaraderie. Members talk, laugh, swap stories and recipes, listen to speakers, and share their struggles and their successes. Many have remarkable stories to tell.

There is Shannon Farrell, a forty-seven-year-old cardiac nurse who found herself, in her mid-thirties, in a downward spiral of health problems including diabetes, Hashimoto's thyroiditis, and severe heart failure. One doctor told her she had fewer than five years to live. Through transitioning to a plant-based diet, Shannon lost eighty-five pounds, reduced her daily medications from twenty-six to just four, reversed almost all of her conditions, and ran her first half marathon this year. "I need to get a new passport photo," she says, "because people don't believe I'm the same person!"

There is David Henderson, who at age sixty-five was overweight and short of breath and felt he was "living on borrowed time." His father and one set of grandparents had had massive heart attacks; the other set of grandparents had had massive strokes. David was sure he was next—until he learned about the power of plant-based nutrition and started to change his diet, "one meal at a time," as he puts it. PBNSG supported him through a sixty-five-pound weight loss. "I have much more energy now," he says, "I used to be out of breath just dragging my trash cart back up my drive. Now I can run up like I was a teenager! Sometimes I ask myself, whose body is this? And all I did was change my diet."

Detroit might seem an unlikely frontier in our country's efforts to stem the tide of obesity, diabetes, heart disease, and other foodborne epidemics. But spend a few days there and you might start thinking differently. A growing crop of plant-based cardiologists, nutritionists, medical centers, and restaurants—including Dr. Kahn's GreenSpace Café, the largest plant-based restaurant in the Midwest—is dedicated to helping people improve their health through the power of whole plant foods.

This quiet revolution is not occurring just in Detroit's wealthy suburbs. Head across the infamous 8 Mile Road and into the recently revitalized downtown and you might run into Akua Woolbright, PhD, a nutritionist who works with Whole Foods Market's Whole Cities Foundation. Woolbright has spent the past three years taking her message to Detroit's diverse communities, speaking at churches, street fairs, beauty salons, and barbershops, and, more recently, in a new teaching kitchen, where every class is filled to capacity.

"People don't want a watered-down message," she says. "They don't just want to hear, 'Eat a few more vegetables.' From my first day here, this community demanded the hard science." What does she tell them? Eat real food. Eat plants. And cut out the processed food that's poisoning you. "You can't keep eating a hot mess and then throw some goji berries on top and think that will make you healthy! To achieve health and wellness, you must make a bold change to a whole foods, plant-based diet. There are no shortcuts."[24]

Woolbright has witnessed similarly powerful results to those reported by her neighbors at PBNSG. People are losing weight, getting off medications, reversing chronic disease, and taking control of their health, many for the first time in their lives. Inspired by these successes, Woolbright and her colleagues at Whole Cities Foundation now train and mentor other advocates to take the message to communities like Chicago's South Side and New Orleans' Ninth Ward.

Detroit is a reminder that in America bad eating habits and their deadly results cut across race, class, and income, afflicting young and old, rich and poor, urban and rural, native and immigrant alike. So it is fitting, perhaps, that a city once considered a microcosm of our nation's deepest problems is discovering, in the nutritional power of real food, a pathway to healing.

Our national health crisis is significant, and it is deeply entangled with our institutions. Industry, government, education, and healthcare each play a part in reinforcing unhealthy patterns. However, the change that is needed will not start at the top. As our friends in Detroit and thousands of others across the country are demonstrating, change starts with individuals who want to be healthy and want to know the truth about how to get there. It starts with people who experience the power of food as medicine and begin to tell other people about it—not just their families and friends, but their doctors, their local restaurants, their children's schools, and their corner stores. Slowly but surely, plant-based whole foods are becoming more widely available, and it's happening because America's consumers are beginning to ask for it. Pioneers like Dr. Ornish and Dr. Esselstyn, among others, have given us the proof of what's possible. It's up to all of us to do our part by embracing our own health potential and encouraging our friends and family to do the same.

꩜ WHOLE FOODIE TAKEAWAYS ꩜

- **Heart disease is not a death sentence**—It has been decisively proven to be preventable and even reversible with whole foods, plant-based diets.
- **Change starts at home**—Don't wait for the medical establishment to catch up. Be a leader in your family and your community.

CHAPTER 6

The Epidemic of Our Time

Demystifying Diabetes

"No disease that can be treated by diet should be treated
with any other means."

— *Maimonides, Medieval Sephardic Jewish Philosopher*

Blindness. Kidney disease. Nerve damage. Amputations. Heart disease. Stroke. Infections. What do all of these have in common? They are all potential complications of one of today's most common chronic diseases: diabetes. As obesity rates have climbed over the past few decades, diabetes rates have escalated dramatically worldwide alongside them. This parallel is no mystery: the World Health Organization lists excess weight gain, being overweight, obesity, and physical inactivity, among other factors, as being directly accountable for the diabetes epidemic.

The statistics on diabetes are simply staggering. More than 29 million Americans are diabetic and 86 million more are prediabetic (meaning that they are likely to be diabetic in ten years or fewer).[1] Most of those people have no idea of this chronic problem lurking inside them. Research suggests that even people with prediabetes may already be suffering negative health consequences.[2] That means more than a hundred million people could be doing long-term damage to their bodies without even knowing it.

Understanding Diabetes

To understand diabetes you need to understand the role of blood sugar. Blood sugar is another term for glucose, the body's preferred source of energy. The food we eat gets broken down into glucose, transported through the bloodstream, and taken into the cells, with help from an essential hormone called insulin. Insulin is produced by the beta cells in our pancreas, and its primary function is to activate insulin receptors in the cells, which allows the glucose to enter the cells from the bloodstream, to then be broken down into energy the body can use. Diabetes refers to a condition in which blood sugar (glucose) cannot get into the cells and as a result starts to build up in the bloodstream.

Neal Barnard, MD, founder of the Physicians Committee for Responsible Medicine, offers a helpful analogy for diabetes. Imagine the cells in our bodies are little houses with doors that need to be opened to let the visiting glucose in. The job of insulin is to act as a key to open those doors and let the glucose into the cell, where it can be turned into energy the body can use. This process can go wrong in two ways. In some cases there is no insulin (no key) to open the door, so the glucose gets stuck outside—this is known as type 1 diabetes, which usually occurs in childhood as a result of an autoimmune response that damages the cells that make insulin. People with type 1 diabetes must take insulin, hence it is often known as *insulin-dependent diabetes*. Type 1 diabetes is less common, accounting for only 5% to 10% of cases.

In the second problematic scenario, which is much more common, the insulin, or key, is present but it is unable to open the door. "It is as if the lock has somehow become jammed and the key no longer works,"[3] writes Barnard. This condition is known as *insulin resistance*, which leads to type 2 diabetes, where glucose builds up in the bloodstream. In this setting the body actually tries to make more insulin (more keys) in an effort to get that door open, but the lock is jammed so none of the keys work. It typically occurs in adulthood, often developing slowly, and is closely correlated with a high-fat diet and weight gain. Today, however, more and more

MY WHOLE FOODIE STORY

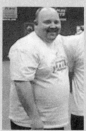 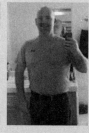

Marty Jenkins, 45, Roseville, California

"Did you know you have diabetes?" The question shocked me. I'd come to Dr. Joel Fuhrman's weeklong Immersion because I wanted to learn more about healthy eating in order to be a better leader in my job at Whole Foods Market. My initial intention was not to change my life or even my health. I knew I was overweight, but didn't really see myself that way. I was a happy person, with a great family, a lovely wife, and a job I enjoyed. I was pretty clueless about my health, but ignorance is bliss, as they say. Until I heard that simple question, and realized, maybe ignorance was not bliss after all! Suddenly my journey became a very personal one.

The bad news didn't stop at diabetes. I had high blood pressure, and I weighed 280 pounds. I had arrived there prepared to learn, but not prepared for seven days of challenging emotions and meals without the things I loved most. I was accustomed to eating meat twice a day, seven days a week. I ate sweets like there was no tomorrow, and drank a six-pack of soda a day. I entered competitive BBQ competitions and made my own BBQ sauce. But now I was invested in making a change. I knew something was wrong, and I had the power to take care of it.

My road to health hasn't been easy, and to be totally honest, I hated the food for about two months until my taste buds changed. People told me that would happen, but I didn't really believe it until one day suddenly the food started to taste amazing. Meals with no salt, no oil, and no processed foods can and will taste good if you give them a chance.

Today I am the same happy man I was before, just much healthier and in control of my life. In only nine months, I lost over ninety pounds, my blood pressure dropped from 156/96 to 115/75, and I'm no longer diabetic, with my blood sugar regularly testing between 70 and 80. I believe in this program because it saved my life.

children are being diagnosed with type 2 diabetes as a by-product of rising childhood obesity.

Many people don't realize that type 2 diabetes is a disease that can be largely prevented or reversed through dietary intervention. Even in those cases where it is not reversible, as well as cases of type 1 diabetes, the severity of the illness can be significantly reduced. Yet most doctors don't take this approach of using nutrition to effectively treat diabetes.

Instead they prescribe medications to lower blood sugar—an approach that has limited value. A large review of randomized clinical trials in the *BMJ* showed that using medications to intensively control blood sugar does not prevent overall death or mitigate some of the other effects of diabetes, such as cardiovascular disease.[4] In fact, another study, published in *The New England Journal of Medicine*, concluded that trying to achieve normal blood sugar in type 2 diabetics through the use of medications actually increased the risk of death.[5] Even efforts to medicate to maintain "tight glycemic control" or keep blood sugar within a certain lower range have been shown to do little to actually prevent the significant complications of diabetes.[6]

The problem with using medications in this way is that they manipulate the markers of disease (the blood sugar numbers) without treating the underlying problem that makes natural insulin ineffective, blocking the locks to the cell doors. The good news is that just as type 2 diabetes is caused by diet and lifestyle choices, it can be improved or even reversed by diet and lifestyle choices. If you want to have "normal" blood sugar numbers, the safest way is to reverse the disease itself by eating a whole foods, plant-based diet.

Pinpointing the Underlying Problem

Many people are convinced that sugar is the problem when it comes to diabetes. Barnard points out that this is an unfortunate mistaken approach. "People think, I've got too much sugar in my blood, so I shouldn't have any sugar in my diet," he explains. "Then they conclude that they should not eat foods like potatoes or bread or pasta or rice that will release carbohydrates, because the carbohydrate will turn to sugar in the blood."[7] Get rid of sugar in the diet, they believe, and the diabetes will improve. Some extend this judgment to all carbohydrates and even fresh fruit (see box, page 118). What people don't seem to understand, Barnard explains, is that "the problem in diabetes isn't the glucose. The body needs glucose as fuel. The problem is that the glucose isn't getting into the cells. It's staying in the blood."[8]

This bears repeating because the misconception is so common: *Diabetes is not a disease caused by consuming too much sugar; it's a disease caused by problems getting sugar into the cells.* That's not to say sugar is a health food or you should add it to your diet; indeed, quite the opposite. Rather, it is to caution you that if you focus only on avoiding sugar or carbohydrates, you will miss the real culprit.

What is the culprit? In 1999, scientists at Yale University used newly available magnetic resonance spectroscopy technology to show a relationship between the buildup of microscopic fat droplets in the cells (intramyocellular lipids) and insulin resistance.[9] It turns out that fat is "jamming the locks" so insulin cannot open the door. The implication of this is clear: diabetes is caused by the high-fat, meat-heavy, high-calorie Western diet, coupled with a sedentary lifestyle.

As further evidence, Dr. Barnard points out that sugar consumption in America leveled off in about 1999 and has been declining ever since, but diabetes cases keep increasing. "The diabetes epidemic tracks the cheese graphs more closely than it tracks the sugar consumption graphs," he says.

So what diet should we follow if we want to prevent or reverse type 2 diabetes? Dr. Barnard is unequivocal. "We can quite confidently now say that the research favoring plant-based diets is overwhelming. Vegetarians and vegans have the least risk of diabetes by far." Any diet that reduces fat and promotes overall weight loss will improve insulin resistance and diabetes. Because diabetes is actually caused by fat, reducing dietary fat intake has a direct impact on the disease, allowing insulin to begin to function again.[10]

Diets that are rich in plant foods and low in animal foods appear to have the most powerful effect in this regard.[11] This is not a new discovery—studies going back to the 1960s reveal a significant correlation between the frequency of meat consumption and rates of diabetes, and show that those eating a vegetarian diet had the lowest rates of the disease.[12] More recently, the enormous Adventist Health Study-2, following ninety-six thousand people, (which we discussed in chapter 3), showed that diabetes prevalence decreased along with people's consumption of animal foods.[13]

Even on a plant-based diet, should diabetics restrict carbohydrate intake? Science does not support this approach. *The American Journal of Clinical Nutrition* has published multiple articles supporting a high-carbohydrate diet with plenty of fiber as not only safe but also actually the diet of choice for diabetics.[14] Of course, we would add that those carbohydrates should come in the form of fruits, vegetables, whole grains, starchy vegetables, and legumes, rather than in the form of refined and processed foods. This, too, is supported by the data: one study showed that simply replacing one-third of a cup of white rice with the same amount of brown rice per day lowered diabetes risk by 16%.[15] Fiber, from fiber-rich plant foods, has also been shown to reduce fasting blood glucose and glycated hemoglobin, another measure of blood sugar.[16] As we have seen, the healthiest populations around the world, with very low rates of diabetes, eat a predominantly whole foods, plant-based diet with a high percentage of carbohydrates—like the Okinawans with their sweet potatoes, or the Nicoyans with their rice and beans.

For those who think low-carb, high-fat, high-animal product diets are better for insulin levels and blood sugar, it is important to note that animal products have been shown to increase insulin levels significantly as well.[17]

Several doctors have put these correlations to the test in clinical settings, showing that type 2 diabetes can be effectively reversed with a low-fat vegan diet.[18] Dr. Barnard is one of them. He conducted a randomized controlled trial in which a low-fat vegan diet was found to be three times more effective than the American Diabetes Association dietary guidelines at controlling

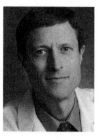

WHOLE FOODIE HERO
Neal Barnard, MD

"If beef is your idea of 'real food for real people,' you'd better live real close to a real good hospital."

Contributions: Barnard is the founding president of the Physicians Committee for Responsible Medicine, committed to treating chronic disease through the promotion of good nutrition and a plant-based diet. PCRM conducts studies, aggregates research, and also advocates for better ethics in research, working to reduce animal experimentation in medical studies.

Fun facts: The year before Barnard went to medical school, his job involved assisting during autopsies. After directly observing the deadly aftermath of America's poor diets—clogged arteries, colon cancer, and other aberrations—he resolved to make an impact on the chronic disease epidemic.

Read this: *Neal Barnard's Program for Reversing Diabetes: The Scientifically Proven System for Reversing Diabetes Without Drugs*

Learn more: pcrm.org

blood sugar. The conventional group reduced its A1c (a measure of blood sugar control) by 0.4 points, on average, which was a good change. But the vegan group reduced its A1c by 1.2 points, which is greater than the effect of typical oral diabetes medicines.[19] These remarkable results illustrate the impact of treatments that don't merely seek to ameliorate symptoms but address the underlying cause of the disease itself. Again, as with heart disease, too often we assume that chronic conditions, once contracted, are irreversible. Never underestimate the body's ability to heal, given the right foods. Diabetes does not have to sentence you to a life of needles and medications. In fact, if you are diabetic and you begin to shift to a whole foods, plant-based diet, you should be sure to talk to your doctor about your blood sugar-lowering medications, because you will likely have to adjust them quite soon.

Blood Sugar, the Glycemic Index, and Your Health

Even if you are not diabetic, you may well have started worrying about your blood sugar, thanks to the recent trend of "blood sugar diets" built around measuring the "glycemic index" or "glycemic load" of certain foods. These measures are supposed to help determine the effect of different foods on

Don't Fear the Fruit!

Some people worry that fruits are a sugary food that should be avoided, causing diabetes and weight gain. These fears are misguided. Yes, fresh fruit contains high levels of fructose, which many people immediately associate with such unhealthy foods as high-fructose corn syrup. However, eating fructose in the form of a whole fruit, with its plentiful fiber, water, and other nutrients, has a very different effect on the body from consuming isolated forms of fructose in sodas, candy, and cookies, all devoid of fiber and nutrients. In fact, fruits have been shown to blunt the effects of other high-glycemic foods on our blood sugar levels.[20]

Fruit is exceptionally good for you! Concerns about fructose should be limited to its refined forms and ignored when it comes to whole fruits. And this is not just our opinion. In fact, in trial after trial, fruit has been shown to have beneficial effects on health—even when consumed in large amounts. In a randomized controlled trial, diabetics showed no negative effects from eating two or more servings of fruit a day. And those who restricted fruit in their diet showed no positive improvement in the disease, prompting researchers to conclude that "intake of fruit should not be restricted" in type 2 diabetics.[21] In other words, no one, not even diabetics, should fear the fruit.

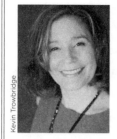

Kevin Trowbridge

WHOLE FOODIE HERO
Brenda Davis, RD

"Vegan diets have not only been vindicated [as nutritionally adequate], they are also being hailed as health heroes, and for good reason. They provide a simple solution for the global epidemic of chronic disease. Well-designed vegan diets afford powerful protection against an imposing list of noncommunicable diseases and serve as safe, economical, and highly effective treatment tools."

Contributions: A registered dietitian and nutritionist who wrote the definitive book on becoming a vegan, Davis has helped people all over the world make the transition to an exclusively plant-based diet with helpful guidance, the latest research, carefully curated recommendations, and expert nutritional information.

Fun facts: When Davis decided to stop eating animal foods, as a result of a crisis of conscience, she did not know one "real live vegetarian."

Read this: *Becoming Vegan: The Complete Reference to Plant-Based Nutrition (Comprehensive Edition,* with Vesanto Melina)

Learn more: brendadavisrd.com

blood sugar and to warn people against foods that create a "spike" or sudden rise in blood sugar. Unfortunately, the picture painted by the glycemic index can be misleading when it comes to health, and its utility has been called into question by the American Diabetes Association, the American Heart Association, and the Academy of Nutrition and Dietetics. *A low glycemic index rating for a food does not mean that that food is a healthy choice.* Increased fat and protein content will bring down a food's glycemic index numbers, but may have many detrimental effects. From a purely commonsense standpoint, when French fries score better than boiled potatoes, and a candy bar appears to be preferable to a carrot, you might want to think twice before basing dietary choices on this rather blunt instrument. It's also important to remember that we usually eat foods in combinations, and one food can change or balance out the glycemic effect of another.

Unfortunately, some have seized on the glycemic index and made a meal out of this small nutritional morsel, drawing unwarranted conclusions about the relationship between a food's ranking on the index and its actual health impact in the body. The glycemic index is only one isolated parameter by which to measure different foods, and it is not a very useful one when it comes to predicting health outcomes. Nor is it necessary when one is following a whole foods, 90+% plant-based diet. There are many numbers a Whole Foodie doesn't have to spend much time worrying about—the glycemic index of foods being one of them!

The Democratization of Chronic Disease

Diabetes is perhaps the most common and chronic of the "diseases of affluence" that are fast becoming the scourge of the developed and developing world. As countries grow wealthier, they have a tendency to get sicker and fatter. Diet-related diseases such as diabetes have jumped America's borders, and are on the rise around the world. A 2012 study in *The Lancet* noted that while we are winning the battle against infectious diseases globally, rates of chronic diseases—heart disease, hypertension, stroke, diabetes, and obesity—are rising.[22]

Diabetes is leading the way. As Barnard explains, "Diabetes is the epidemic of our time, and this epidemic that has been growing in America is now growing worldwide. We are seeing it in India; we are seeing it in China. We are seeing massive increases in diabetes rates pretty much everywhere that you have greater affluence."[23]

If the great challenge of the twentieth century was to turn the tide against deadly infectious diseases such as cholera, smallpox, typhus, and yellow fever, then it certainly looks as if the great challenge of the twenty-first century will be to turn the tide against the chronic diseases that are running rampant across the globe as incomes rise and Western-style food consumption skyrockets. This will take a change of diet, but also a change of mind-set. As Dr. Garth Davis writes, "In contrast [to infectious diseases], an individual can all but eliminate the risk of most chronic diseases through a healthy diet and lifestyle. My medical colleagues still put their faith in pills and surgeries, the tools that were developed for—and triumphed against—infectious disease and traumatic injury. The diet they recommend corresponds to this outdated worldview as well."[24]

Ironically, our current unhealthy state of affairs is also a sign of something deeply positive. It speaks of a world in which more and more people are actually becoming affluent. More of us are living, and eating, as kings and queens once did—but that's not necessarily a good thing! There was a time when diseases of affluence were limited to a very small segment of the population—the rich. Being fat or portly or obese was a status symbol, as was the regular consumption of meat. Everyone else, for the most part, was poor and thin. The poor and working class used meat and animal products as condiments or for occasional feasts, not as the main dish at every meal. They couldn't afford to do otherwise.

In the modern industrialized era, that pattern has been almost completely reversed. Incomes have gone up, and industrialized food production, together with generous government subsidies, has dramatically lowered the prices of meat, eggs, and dairy products, as well as highly processed foods. Now even the poor can suffer the sicknesses once reserved for the rich. It seems that the powerful economic engines of modernity have unwittingly democratized diseases once reserved for an elite few. In the process of making the diet of the rich cheap, we've also made the diseases of the rich common.

While no developed country has yet been successful at significantly reversing the diseases of affluence, there have been signs of progress in America—among the middle and upper classes. New research suggests that obesity is now leveling off in youth from a higher socioeconomic background. Unfortunately, it is still increasing in youth from impoverished backgrounds.[25] Some have suggested this is because healthier foods, particularly fresh fruits and vegetables, are now more expensive than hamburgers, fries, and other processed fare. When processed, refined foods and animal products are so cheap and ubiquitous, the former diet of the poor seems more difficult and expensive by comparison—even though experts have pointed out that eating whole foods and plants is actually still inexpensive. It seems we need another kind of democratization—the democratization of knowledge regarding healthy eating habits. And we need it urgently—so the onetime diseases of affluence don't become the bane of the developing world. With the spread of good nutritional information, and the support to act on it, we can truly enter a new era—free of both the infectious *and* the chronic diseases that inhibit our global health potential.

➣ WHOLE FOODIE TAKEAWAYS ❧

• **Diabetes is preventable and reversible**—If you've developed or are at risk for type 2 diabetes, you're not sentenced to a life on medications. A whole foods, plant-based diet has been proven to prevent, and in many cases, reverse the disease.

• **Type 2 diabetes is not caused by sugar and carbohydrate foods**—It's caused by a diet heavy in fat and animal foods. Avoiding refined sugar is always a good idea, but don't cut out whole carbohydrate foods or fruits—cut back on animal foods instead.

CHAPTER 7

The Great Grain Robbery

Rethinking the Low-Carb Trend

"The best lies contain a kernel of truth."

—*T. Colin Campbell, The Low-Carb Fraud*

"I'll have the bacon cheeseburger, but hold the bun."

"I don't eat grains; they make you fat."

"Don't blame the butter for what the bread did."

Maybe you've heard statements like this from family, friends, or acquaintances. Maybe you've even uttered them yourself. One of the most popular and powerful dietary trends of the past couple of decades is the "low-carb" movement, which has inspired millions of Americans to shun carbohydrate foods.

Technically carbohydrates are sugar molecules found in many different foods, particularly sugars, starches, and fibers. They are one of the human body's primary sources of energy, and play an important role in any healthy, optimal diet. While carbohydrates are an element of most foods, especially plants, the colloquial term *carbs* is commonly used to refer to foods like sugars, grains and grain products, and starchy vegetables. From Atkins to South Beach to the Zone to today's best-selling authors like Gary Taubes, Nina Teicholz, and Mark Hyman, popular diets have portrayed these foods as the cause of myriad health problems, from obesity to diabetes to brain diseases. They encourage people to cut out grains, starchy vegetables, and sometimes beans and other legumes, while eating more protein, in the form of animal foods and fat. Attracting millions, these diets have captured a surprisingly large mindshare.

How did America conclude that carbs are the root of all dietary evil? Is rejecting foods like rice, wheat, potatoes, or corn a sound decision? Is it scientific? As with many dietary movements, there are some important kernels of truth amid the claims of the low-carb advocates; there are also plenty of misleading notions. How do we sort the wheat from the chaff when it comes to these ancient foods that have long formed the bulk of human diets?

Whole Grains and Half-Truths

Bread, beans, cookies, corn, rice, cupcakes, oatmeal, yams, potatoes, corn syrup, pasta, candy, table sugar. If you eat a strict low-carb diet, all of those foods will be off the menu, or at least make only rare appearances. Do you see the problem here? Some of these foods are not like the others. Yes, they may all share a common macronutrient, carbohydrates, but the focus on that alone obscures the much more important distinction that is at the heart of this book's dietary philosophy: the difference between whole foods and highly processed foods.

The low-carb people have one thing right: highly processed, refined carbohydrate foods spell disaster for health. Humans love carbohydrates— they are the body's preferred energy source. Approximately 50% of the calories Americans eat come from this food category,[1] and that is actually on the low side of USDA recommendations.[2] Unfortunately, we love carbs so much that we've come up with endless delicious delivery systems for the sugars and starches we crave. We subject them to industrial processes, manipulating and refining them until something comes out that no longer resembles the original food at all.

Like all processed foods, highly refined carbohydrates lack fiber and healthful micronutrients, while delivering a condensed load of calories. The body essentially can't distinguish them from white sugar (empty calories devoid of any nutritional value), and treats them just as poorly, leading to weight gain and a host of related problems. The growing recognition of the dangers of highly processed foods in general, many of which are in fact refined carbohydrates, has helped drive the low-carb movement forward.

"Carbs are bad" is, in this sense, a half-truth. Yes, highly processed carbs are something we would all do well to avoid. But in the name of protecting people against the evils of refined carbohydrates, the low-carb movement has created an enormous amount of confusion about the role of unprocessed carbohydrate foods, robbing millions of Americans of the tremendous proven health benefits of whole grains, beans, and starchy vegetables. Furthermore, it has encouraged those same people to increase their consumption of animal foods, with all its well-documented health risks.

There is a universe of difference between a box of sugary processed oat-flour cereal and a bowl of steel-cut oats, between the white flour in a cupcake and the whole grains in traditional bread. All are high-carbohydrate foods. But the purveyors of low-carb diets too often act as if the term *carbohydrate* were synonymous with refined, processed foods loaded with extra fat and sugar. Both in popular diet books and supposedly rigorous scientific studies comparing the effects of different diets on health, authors often don't distinguish clearly enough between foods in whole forms and the much less nutritious processed versions. Yes, a control group in a study may eat carbohydrates instead of fats, but what kind of carbs? If it's cookies and cupcakes, we shouldn't be surprised when they don't fare so well. That answer makes all the difference when it comes to the results of the study, just as it does when it comes to your health and the food on your plate.

The history of the modern low-carb movement can be traced to the outsize influence of Dr. Robert Atkins and the empire he created, beginning with his 1972 book, *Dr. Atkins' Diet Revolution*. In it he advises people to shun carbs, and eat more protein and fat. He encourages people to eat animal foods in abundance, including butter, lard, and bacon, and discourages fruits and green vegetables.

Despite finding little support in the medical or nutritional communities, Atkins' controversial book, and its 1992 follow-up, sold more than fifteen million copies, one of the best-selling diet books ever.

Atkins coined the phrase *low carb*, and his success likely inspired the current glut of similar diets. Some have grown more sophisticated and evolved their overall message from Atkins, but they still contain many of the basic elements. They tell us to eat more fats and protein, including more meat, and to beware of carbohydrates.

There is also a consistent effort to frame sugar as the primary problem in the Standard American Diet, almost as if sugar's sacrifice could redeem every other dietary vice. This "sacrificial nutrient" approach is a common theme in

MY WHOLE FOODIE STORY

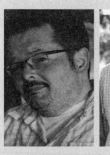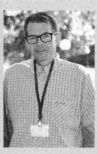

Frank Schuck, 45, Seattle, Washington
"Dads don't run." The words of my eight-year-old son stuck in my head and wouldn't leave me alone. At more than three hundred pounds, I didn't feel so bad, but I couldn't deny that I wasn't able to do the things I would have liked to do, like run with my kids. In October 2013, at the age of 41, that all began to change. I was fortunate enough to attend Dr. McDougall's Immersion in Santa Rosa, California, and it turned out to be a life changer for me.

Before that week, I had been the first to make jokes about vegetarians and vegans. My job is specialty coordinator for Whole Foods Market in the Northwest, which means I'm in charge of cheese, chocolate, beer, wine, and spirits—all the sinful things! But the Immersion was an eye-opener and it inspired me to adopt a plant-based diet.

I now weigh 154 pounds and have kept that weight off for going on three years. I'm literally half the man I used to be! I won't say it's easy to lose weight—it's not. The path is easy; keeping on it is the hard part. But it's worth it.

I'm a "starchivore"—which means 60% of my calories come from starches. I love starches—like potatoes and corn and rice. I don't the diet world. Just give up X, we are told, and you can freely eat everything else from A to Z. If X happens to be something you like but is not your favorite food, sometimes the trade-off seems worth it. Hence, the attraction of the Atkins diet and its successors isn't necessarily in the avoidance of carbs. It is in the welcome justification to enjoy butter, cheese, bacon, steak, and other animal foods without guilt. Unfortunately, healthy nutrition is a much more holistic process and doesn't work this way. As much as refined sugar may deserve crucifixion, it can't die for all our dietary sins!

eat anything processed, only whole plant foods. For me, one of the keys is to do batch cooking. On the weekends, when I'm with the kids, I make my own bread, or cook large pots of beans and rice, so it's there and it's easy. I think that's the hard part for people who radically change their diets—the convenience factor. They think, "I've got to go to work. I don't have time." But the fact is, if you have time to sit and watch *Survivor* for an hour or so, you have time to cook enough food to get you through the week. I've even gone to friends' homes and done batch cooking for them so they see how easy it is. Once you have the staples ready and in your fridge, you can make so many different menu items. Learning to cook without oil was a challenge at first, but now I have many other options.

My family doesn't eat exactly like I do. But we all dine together, and our base meal is always vegan. For example, we'll have baked potatoes or spaghetti or tacos, and what I put on them may be different from what my wife or kids do. They might have cheese or bacon, while I'll have beans and vegetables. I've noticed, over time, however, that my kids have started to change their habits, just through association with me.

People always ask me, What do you miss? Is it bacon or cheese? But the truth is, I don't feel like I've lost anything. I've gained so much—gained extra years of my life; gained energy and vitality. If someone says, "Here, eat some bacon," I'd rather not, because I'd rather keep the things I've gained. And now my son knows that dads *do* run. I'm even a little faster than he is.

Even critics acknowledge that low-carb diets can result in weight loss. When the body has fewer carbs to burn, it begins to burn fat, a condition known as ketosis. This means that your body burns fat as fuel instead of glucose, its preferred energy source, and that can result in temporary weight loss. People often feel nauseated after some time on this diet, which leads to lower calorie intake over time, further increasing weight loss. However, low-carb diets are notoriously hard to stay on (perhaps due to the lack of truly satiating foods like whole grains, beans, and starchy vegetables) and so weight loss is often temporary, as people "fall off the wagon."

While many low-carb diets are promoted as a healthy means of losing weight, they are in fact associated with higher all-cause mortality in both men and women.[3] Indeed, you would be hard-pressed to find any significant scientific evidence that an Atkins-like diet has good health outcomes over the long term, and it has certainly not been shown to reverse chronic disease. Even temporary weight loss can be matched and probably far exceeded over the long term by a healthier whole foods, plant-based diet that includes whole grains, beans, and starchy vegetables.

Don't Fear the Starch

"All large populations of trim, healthy people, throughout human history, have obtained the bulk of their calories from starch," declares the man on stage, as several hundred people listen closely in the packed auditorium. Dr. John McDougall is addressing a crowd of doctors, health professionals, and health seekers who gather twice a year near his home in Santa Rosa, California, for an Advanced Study Weekend to learn the latest on the benefits of a whole foods, plant-based diet.

For several decades McDougall has been sounding the alarm about the dangers of the Standard American Diet and placing particular emphasis on the benefits of starch-based carbohydrates as essential to human health. "Examples of thriving people include Japanese and Chinese in Asia eating sweet potatoes, buckwheat, and/or rice, Incas in South America eating potatoes, Mayans and

Aztecs in Central America eating corn, and Egyptians in the Middle East eating wheat," he explains. "Over the past century there has been an escalating trend in Western societies of people abandoning starchy plant foods for low-carbohydrate meat and dairy foods. A worldwide epidemic of obesity, heart disease, diabetes, and cancer has followed this dietary change."[4]

In the popular press, Dr. Dean Ornish has often been cast as the dietary opposite to Dr. Atkins, but in truth, McDougall is probably the better adversary, if simply because he has such a deep passion for the starch foods that are so often decried by low-carb advocates. This passion arose from his own experience, in medicine and in life. Afflicted by a rare stroke at the very young age of eighteen, for which doctors had little explanation (and which still affects his movement today), he realized that he was going to have to seek out answers on his own. After medical school he ended up in Hawaii, his patients the thousands of laborers in the sugar plantations and their families.

Here McDougall soon encountered the essential contradiction of modern medicine—that while he could help his patients with infections and injuries, there was little he could do to ameliorate the chronic conditions— diabetes, arthritis, obesity, heart disease, and cancer—that they were suffering from. And his curious mind noticed an important truth about his patients in Hawaii—that while you might expect chronic disease to be correlated with aging, the younger generations were in fact much worse off than the older ones. The reason was not mysterious. Younger generations had increasingly adopted American-style eating habits. They were fatter and sicker. What did the older generations eat? Rice and vegetables were the foundation of their diet, while their children and grandchildren were adding meat, dairy, and processed foods to their plates at high rates.

McDougall's search for answers led him back to the library. He combed through medical and scientific journals for more information on the nutritional patterns he had witnessed in his own patients, and soon amassed a significant body of research showing that a diet based on starch foods, combined with fruits and vegetables, led to optimal health outcomes largely free of chronic disease.

As McDougall discovered, in stark contrast to the current cultural concern about carbs, many civilizations had based their entire diets around starch foods. All of the Blue Zones, as we explained in a previous chapter, relied on corn, yams, or grains for a large percentage of calories—with impressive health outcomes. Those populations experience low obesity, low dementia, and low chronic disease—quite the opposite of what carb-phobic authors would have you believe. As McDougall writes in his book *The Starch Solution: Eat the Foods You Love, Regain Your Health, and Lose the Weight for Good!*, "Throughout civilization and around the world, six foods have provided our primary fuel— barley, corn, millet, potatoes, rice, and wheat."[5] Beans, sweet potatoes, and oats could probably be made honorary members of this list.

Our bodies easily and efficiently use the energy contained in starch. We break down complex carbohydrates over time into simple sugars, providing sustained energy for living. Perhaps most importantly, starch foods can be very satiating (see chapter 2). As a result we tend to consume fewer calories when we adopt a whole foods diet that is rich in starches. These foods also provide us with a particular type of fiber, resistant starch that has all kinds of intestinal benefits. They are full of vitamins and minerals, a source of both nutrients and energy.

McDougall has little patience for vegan or plant-based diets that emphasize other vegetables at the expense of starches. "People try to eat diets centered around kale, broccoli, cauliflower, celery, and so on," he declares, "and it doesn't work! You must have starch as the center of your meal plan. Once you get the starch foods as the centerpiece, then everything works."[6]

In his research McDougall stumbled upon the work of several people who seemed to confirm his intuitions about the power of carbohydrate-rich diets, including Walter Kempner, a German refugee who conducted research at Duke University in the 1930s and got remarkable results treating patients with his famous Rice Diet. While his prescription of white rice, sugar, fruit, fruit juices, vitamins, and iron[7] is not a diet we'd recommend to anyone with better options, Kempner's dramatic results—which included the reversal of diabetes, heart disease, obesity, arthritis, hypertension, and more—run strongly counter to conventional low-carb theories.

Another significant influence was Denis Burkitt, an Irish doctor who spent much of his career in Uganda after World War II. His contributions include raising awareness of the important role of fiber (found only in plant foods). He recognized that the diseases present in African rural hospitals were very different from Western ones, and he hypothesized that the high fiber in the African diet of the time might play a role in protecting people from common Western ailments, which were rare in Uganda and, in fact, all of Africa. His conviction was that many chronic diseases were entirely preventable, and fiber intake was key—which he summed up in a simple equation: Big stools = small hospitals. Small stools = big hospitals.

Nathan Pritikin (see chapter 5) was perhaps McDougall's greatest nutritional influence. In 1978 someone gave him a set of Pritikin's lectures on audiotape. For this young doctor asking serious questions about the state of the American nutritional orthodoxy, Pritikin's example was like finding gold— an important confirmation of his own experience in the sugar plantations of Hawaii. Four decades later McDougall has gone on to help thousands of patients get off the chronic disease train, all while publishing books, papers, and newsletters, and providing an educational platform to enable experts and laypeople alike to explore the power of food as medicine.

Indeed, his center in Santa Rosa has served as something of an incubator for the larger plant-based nutrition movement for several decades. In addition to his Advanced Study Weekends, which combine education with inspiration, he welcomes a steady flow of people to his weeklong intensives. A 2014 study published in *Nutrition Journal* tracked more than sixteen hundred patients who had attended these intensives, and found that average weight loss in just one week was three pounds, average cholesterol reduction was 22 mg/dL, and nearly 90% of patients were able to get off blood pressure and diabetic medications.[8] And McDougall proudly emphasizes that participants get to eat as much as they like during the week. The overflowing buffet has become famous, with many recipes straight from the kitchen of Mary McDougall, his wife and collaborator. Front and center at every meal are whole grains and starchy vegetables.

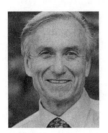

WHOLE FOODIE HERO
John McDougall, MD

"The fat you eat is the fat you wear."

Contributions: In addition to his work with thousands of patients over the years, Dr. McDougall has provided invaluable educational opportunities through his conferences, immersions, workshops, intensives, and other activities designed to spread the word about the power of starch-based eating.

Fun facts: Dr. McDougall met his wife, Mary, in an operating room when he was in medical school and she was a surgical nurse. These days their work together has moved from the operating table to the dinner table, with Mary McDougall creating many of the delicious, healthy recipes offered in Dr. McDougall's programs and books.

Read this: *The Starch Solution: Eat the Foods You Love, Regain Your Health, and Lose the Weight for Good!*

Learn more: drmcdougall.com

Grappling with Grains and Gluten

Walk into any grocery store these days and briefly examine the row upon row of foods proclaiming themselves "gluten-free," and you would be excused for thinking that we are in the midst of a nationwide epidemic of disease and that gluten is the proven culprit. While today's low-carb diets and philosophies build on Atkins' approach, their arguments often emphasize gluten as playing a key role in making Americans fat, sick, and stupid.

So what is gluten? As the comedian Jimmy Kimmel demonstrated in a hilarious and revealing 2014 video, even many people who don't eat it don't know what it is. Gluten is a mixture of proteins found in wheat and a number of other grains, including barley and rye. It's the substance that makes bread and grains chewy. If you've ever kneaded dough, it's what gives it that elastic feeling.

A number of books, including *Wheat Belly* by Dr. William Davis and *Grain Brain* by Dr. David Perlmutter, have risen to the top of best-seller lists by blaming wheat in general and gluten specifically for America's chronic diseases, obesity rates, and even mental disorders—from Alzheimer's to schizophrenia to autism. Davis, a cardiologist, goes so far as to claim that wheat has killed more people than all wars combined. Perlmutter declares that gluten sensitivity "represents one of the greatest and most underrecognized health threats to humanity."[9] This kind of dramatic hyperbole is not uncommon in the "war on wheat" subculture. Is it justified?

The first important truth to acknowledge is that some people have celiac disease and as a result are highly gluten intolerant. When they eat gluten, they suffer damage to the small intestine (visible on a biopsy) that can lead to a host of ills, including unhealthy weight loss and the inability to absorb nutrients. This is a genetic autoimmune disorder, and estimates of the population affected tend to be low, around 1%.[10] However, that is still several million people who need to be very aware of the dangers of ingesting gluten. For celiac sufferers, a gluten-free diet is essential, although there is no reason these people should not consume other healthy carbohydrate foods like nonglutenous whole grains and starchy vegetables.

The question then arises: How much of the explosion of concern about gluten sensitivity in the rest of the population is legitimate? In recent years nutrition experts have come to recognize that there is indeed a population of individuals that is sensitive to gluten and/or allergic to wheat but who do not have celiac disease. For these people, ingesting gluten may trigger physical symptoms such as abdominal pain, bloating, diarrhea, constipation, bone or joint pain, headaches, and fatigue. There is some evidence that their sensitivities can affect their mood and mental state as well. Again, estimates as to the size of this cohort are relatively low, around 1% or perhaps slightly higher.[11] Unfortunately, these individuals have often gone undiagnosed in the medical system.

These two populations—celiac sufferers and gluten-sensitive people—do not, however, come anywhere near to accounting for America's great gluten freak out. The number claiming either gluten intolerance or an allergy to wheat far exceeds the actual estimates of sufferers (which would add up to little more than 2%). Researchers estimate that as many as 30% of American adults are choosing to cut down on or avoid gluten, and an even higher percentage believe gluten-free foods are healthier options.[12] Are these people misguided? In one double-blind, controlled Italian study, patients claiming nonceliac gluten intolerance were tested, under very rigorous conditions, and 86% were clearly shown to have nothing of the sort.[13]

Interestingly, we've observed that often, when people who believe themselves to be gluten sensitive try a whole foods, plant-based diet, they feel better regardless of whether they restrict gluten (possibly incriminating the other unhealthy foods they have now stopped eating as the true cause of their symptoms).

How Grains Are Processed and Why It Matters

To understand the processing journey that takes a health-promoting whole grain and turns it into a health risk, let's use the example of wheat. To obtain the edible wheat grain or kernel, the inedible husk is removed from the grain after harvesting. A wheat kernel is made up of the outer layer of bran, the inner layer of endosperm, and a seed germ. Each element brings nutritional benefits to the table—the endosperm is made up of mostly starchy carbohydrates; the germ is the part of the kernel involved in reproduction and contains a powerful mix of vitamins, minerals, and nutrients; and the bran contains the helpful fiber that is so important to the overall nutritional package of plant foods.

In a whole grain food, the entire wheat kernel is used. If it is whole grain flour, the entire kernel is milled, so it still has the nutrients and fiber. That is far preferable to a refined grain or white flour, where only the endosperm is ground, leaving a starchy carbohydrate with some nutrients, but without many of the other nutritional elements that make a whole grain a nutritional powerhouse. Plus refined grains are often combined with other unhealthy ingredients, such as sugar and oil. There is evidence that while whole grain

Unfortunately, the current wave of concern over gluten leads too many people in unhealthy directions. Either they load up on gluten-free versions of their favorite foods, which are often more processed than the originals, packed with sugar, fat, and highly refined gluten-free flours, or they head on over to the low-carb camp, and shun all grains, glutenous or otherwise. But science to date has consistently revealed impressive health benefits associated with whole grains.[14] *Whole grains are healthy foods.* One recent study in the *BMJ* shows how whole grain consumption is associated with a reduction in cancer, heart disease, respiratory disease, and infectious disease, including a 17%-reduction in all-cause mortality.[15] Another study that reviewed the findings of twelve studies involving eight hundred thousand people over four decades found that the higher the consumption of whole grains, the lower

consumption is associated with less abdominal fat in adults, *refined grain consumption is just the opposite.*[19]

Read food labels carefully when buying grain-based products. Some foods are labeled as containing whole grains, but check the percentage before you put them in your shopping basket—they may not be 100% whole grain. Others use terms like *multigrain*, which simply means that they contain more than one type of flour—and they can all be refined. Even those that do actually use whole wheat or whole grain ingredients too often add plenty of other questionable substances—enough to make the whole package a nutritional no-no.

This brings us back, once again, to our first rule: choose whole foods instead of highly processed foods. For example, choose brown rice over white, or whole wheat pasta over refined alternatives. Choose whole grain breads, ideally made with coarse-ground flour and with a high ratio of fiber to carbohydrates (see "Tips for Reading Food Labels" on page 162 for more advice on choosing breads). As always, grains in their intact form are the healthiest choice. Remember, *the closer a grain is to its original intact whole form, the more nutritional benefits it will likely bestow.*

the death rate—a reduction in risk of 25% for heart disease and 15% for cancer.[16] Daily consumption of three portions of whole grains has even been shown to be so effective at lowering blood pressure that it could decrease the incidence of coronary artery disease by 15% and stroke by 25%.[17] Whole grain consumption has been demonstrated to increase insulin sensitivity, thus reducing the risk of diabetes.[18] These are just a few of the many results over the years that have confirmed, and reconfirmed, the nutritional benefits of whole grains. Indeed, the positive health evidence for whole grains continues to grow, despite the claims of fad diet books. It would be a travesty to see people continue to shun a whole host of healthy foods in order to hedge against a condition that they most likely don't have!

We hope evidence like this convinces you not to fear wheat or other glutenous grains in whole food forms, no matter what you may read or hear. Unless you are one of the 2% to 3% with celiac disease, wheat allergy, or gluten sensitivity, you can embrace glutenous whole grains and whole grain products, including wheat, and enjoy all their benefits. Gluten is not the source of all dietary evil, nor will avoiding it be the single dietary miracle cure to all that ails you. If you decide to avoid gluten, simply choose nonglutenous whole grains, like brown rice, oats, millet, quinoa, or buckwheat. And don't make the mistake of thinking a "gluten-free" label is a ticket to health. Gluten-free cookies are still cookies. With so many unhealthy processed foods being produced in gluten-free forms, the same principles apply to a gluten-free diet as to any optimal diet. Choose whole foods, mostly plants.

An Inflammatory Conversation

Today's scaremongering around wheat is not just about extra calories, or the pulverized grains, or the lack of fiber, or the added fats and sugars in some forms. It's also about the boogeyman of "inflammation." In some diet books about wheat and grains, it's as if the unseen evil of chronic inflammation is lurking in our body ready to attack, and all it ever needs is a smidgen of wheat! The idea is that wheat is high glycemic, which might cause higher blood sugar, and higher blood sugar might lead to inflammation, which might lead to various long-term health problems. Here again we have to tread carefully and follow the science. There is little evidence that genuinely whole wheat foods result in inflammation. In fact, quite the opposite. Diets high in whole grains have consistently been shown to reduce levels of systemic inflammation.[20] On the other hand, animal foods, which are what many people tend to load up on when they reduce consumption of grains and other high-carbohydrate foods, have been shown to increase inflammation.[21]

The fear of wheat runs dangerously close to scaremongering and pseudoscience. The Grim Reaper of inflammation is not lurking behind every grain (unless, of course, actual allergies are involved, since any food you are allergic to will cause inflammation). As Dr. Michael Greger explains, "If someone says whole wheat is inflammatory, then show me a single study anywhere in a nonceliac disease population that says that. I don't know of any. But of course, if you are talking about refined grains, it's different. People who think they can live on vegan donuts are kidding themselves."[22] A healthy, whole foods, plant-based diet that includes whole grains is not going to negatively impact your overall blood sugar or inflammation levels. Likely it will do just the opposite.

Here's the bottom line: The rhetoric over grains is overblown, indiscriminate, and, well, inflammatory. It has thrown out the baby of whole grains with the bathwater of more processed, refined versions. Next time your friend orders that bacon cheeseburger without the bun, "because carbs make you fat," you'll know that yes, refined white flour buns probably will make you fat, and sick as well, but so will the processed meat burger. Whole carbohydrate foods, however, do quite the opposite. So go ahead and order a big portion of brown rice and vegetables, or even a bean burger on a whole wheat bun, knowing that whole grains are consistently associated with good health, weight loss, and longer life.

⌒ WHOLE FOODIE TAKEAWAYS ⌒

• **Carbs do not make you fat or sick, so long as they are whole foods**—Know the difference between unhealthy processed carbs and healthy whole grains and starchy vegetables.

• **Whole grains, starchy vegetables, and legumes should be the base of your diet**—These foods are consistently associated with better health and greater satiety.

• **Gluten intolerance and celiac disease are rare**—Unless you are part of that 2% to 3% of the population, there is no reason you should avoid glutenous whole grains like wheat.

CHAPTER 8

The Caveman Cometh

Promises and Pitfalls of the Paleo Diet

"The past is our definition. We may strive, with good reason, to escape
it, or to escape what is bad in it, but we will escape it only by adding
something better to it."

—*Wendell Berry*

What do yoga mats, flip-flops, and Subway buns have in common? Until
very recently, the chemical azodicarbonamide. In 2016 the sandwich giant,
along with several other fast-food chains, made headlines when they
announced (quietly) that they would remove this "dough conditioner"
from their breads. There's no doubt this is good news for their customers,
since azodicarbonamide has been linked to asthma and cancer, but it begs
the question, what on earth was it doing there in the first place? One might
ask the same about countless other chemicals that show up in our food.
Indeed, the additives, preservatives, artificial flavorings, and various other
compounds that comprise the ingredient lists of today's processed foods can
make one's head spin—a veritable chemistry set in every box, bottle, breast,
bun, wing, fry, flake, and Happy Meal. It's enough to make anyone long for a
simpler time when food was, well, food.

And many do. In response to growing awareness of the excesses of
industrialized food, more and more people are searching for an alternative.
Some look back a few hundred years before modern food-distribution
systems brought the world's bounty to our doorsteps. Some harken back to a

pretechnological era when the pace of life was less frenzied. Some decry the modern trend of urbanization and return to the land. Natural and organic foods; locavore; slow food; farm to table—all of these are movements born of food culture's nostalgia for its lost past and many legitimate concerns about today's industrial food systems. But some take that sentiment to a whole different level, and go Paleo.

Michael Pollan likes to say, "Don't consume anything that your great-grandmother wouldn't recognize as food." Paleo, one of today's most popular diet trends, sees that basic concept and raises Pollan a few hundred millennia. It says, don't eat anything that a caveman wouldn't recognize as food.

Paleo stands for *Paleolithic Diet*, a concept that emerged in the 1970s, gained traction in the 1980s thanks to S. Boyd Eaton and Melvin Konner's paper of the same name, and was popularized in the early twenty-first century by best-selling author Loren Cordain and a rapidly growing tribe of adherents. While for some, going Paleo can include many behaviors that may reflect a Paleolithic lifestyle—like running for short intense bursts (akin to escaping predators), squatting rather than sitting to defecate (you can even buy a special toilet accessory called a Squatty Potty), or (for the more extreme) giving blood regularly to approximate the occasional wounds our ancestors must have suffered—it is generally seen as an approach to eating, and for our purposes we'll leave the other lifestyle behaviors aside and focus on the dietary recommendations.

The basic premise of the Paleo diet, as Cordain puts it, is that "Nature determined what our bodies needed thousands of years before civilization developed, before people started farming and raising domesticated livestock."[1] Paleo advocates believe that our bodies have not significantly changed since the Paleolithic era, otherwise known as the Stone Age or the prehistoric era, which began about 2.6 million years ago. This was the era in which hominids lived as hunter-gatherers and began to use basic stone tools. Anatomically modern humans arrived on the scene during this period, around two hundred thousand years ago. The end of the Paleolithic era is marked by the full-scale adoption of agriculture, and the beginning of more complex human settlements, around ten to twelve thousand years ago.

Modern Paleo diets vary a great deal among practitioners. In general, however, they focus on foods like lean grass-fed meat or wild-caught fish (that approximate what we might have hunted or caught) and fruits, vegetables, seeds, and nuts (that approximate what might have been gathered). They eschew foods that they see as being born out of agriculture, like grains, legumes, and starchy vegetables, and they reject most highly processed foods, particularly refined carbohydrates (though, curiously, not certain vegetable oils). They also are suspicious of dairy foods, arguing that only a relatively small percentage of the human population has adapted to tolerate these in more recent history.

Paleo diets are close cousins of the low-carb, high-protein diets discussed in the previous chapter. However, they deserve to be considered on their own terms, both nutritionally and philosophically. Nutritionally, there are certainly some things to like about the Paleo approach—and some overlaps with the Whole Foods Diet—but there are some causes for concern as well. Philosophically, there are some questions that bear closer scrutiny. Even if we knew exactly what our Paleolithic ancestors ate (and we don't), even if Paleo devotees were right in all their claims about our past (and they aren't), and even if we could eat exactly the same type of food as our ancestors (and we can't), there are still serious questions about whether it is the ideal diet for humans today.

The Upsides of Paleo

There are many things to like about the Paleo diet. First and foremost, unlike many food fads of the last few decades, Paleo is resolutely focused on real, whole foods, which are beneficial for health. We have seen again and again the evidence that highly processed foods—sweetened cereals; oily, salty snacks; sugary candy and baked goods; calorie-packed sodas—are not doing any health favors. In fact, Paleo has made one of the two central tenets of the Whole Foods Diet its own—*eat whole foods instead of processed foods.*

Undoubtedly, this is one reason many people feel so much better and lose weight when they adopt a Paleo diet, especially at first. Suddenly they cut out most processed foods from their diet—and if they're anywhere close to the average American, those could account for up to 70% of their previous food choices. Instead they eat primarily real food, maybe for the first time in their lives. It's not surprising that they experience a dramatic difference in health and well-being.

What are those processed foods being replaced with? In part, a larger percentage of animal foods, in the form of eggs, fish, meat, and even organ meats—a concerning direction that we'll discuss in a moment. However, people who adopt a Paleo diet are also encouraged to follow another central tenet of the Whole Foods Diet, and increase their consumption of fruits and vegetables—another reason, no doubt, that people often report positive results when they make the transition. Cut out processed foods and eat more fruits and vegetables—that's a good foundation for any diet.

A third positive about Paleo is its cautious approach toward dairy foods. Dr. Cordain accurately states that "we are the only species on the planet to consume another animal's milk throughout our adult lives. Humans don't have a nutritional requirement for the milk of another species, nor do any other mammals."[2] If you choose to include dairy in your Whole Foods Diet, we recommend doing so in limited quantities. Most Americans consume far too much dairy, and Paleo offers a healthy corrective to this tendency.

The Downsides of Paleo

For all its benefits, in the form of real foods and healthy fruits and veggies, Paleo's downsides are concerning. They start with its conviction that animal foods—in the form of meat, fish, and eggs—should play a central role in one's diet. We have already laid out the serious long-term health concerns raised by an overreliance on animal foods, and the chronic diseases that are associated with such diets (see page 63). A whole foods, plant-based diet need not be vegan or vegetarian, but relying on meat and other animal foods to fill up more than 50% of one's calories, as some in the Paleo camp suggest, is not an evidence-based health choice. Most Americans eat far too much meat already.

Paleo advocates rightly emphasize choosing lean, pastured meats and wild-caught seafood over today's factory-farmed, feedlot fare, pumped full of corn, antibiotics, and hormones. And many warn against processed meats, pointing out that cavemen certainly did not eat lunch meats, hot dogs, and salami—a category of foods recently designated as carcinogenic by the World Health Organization. However, too many adherents unfortunately seem to consider Paleo simply synonymous with meat, and consider their new "evolved" diet a meal ticket to unlimited bacon.

Another problem with eating too much meat and other animal foods is that they tend to crowd out other good things from our diet. Healthy plant foods suddenly become less important when you build a food culture around meat. Even though fruits and vegetables may play a significant role on the plates of some Paleo adherents, they seem to be an afterthought for too many. With the Whole Foods Diet, we take the opposite approach. Some occasional pastured meat or wild-caught fish may have a place on your plate, but it should never be so prominent that it takes space away from whole plant foods.

The other significant downside of Paleo diets is what they leave off the plate altogether: whole grains, starchy vegetables, and beans and other legumes. These foods are rejected primarily because of the idea that they were not part of the human diet before the advent of agriculture, although some of the common low-carb concerns about their healthfulness tend to creep into Paleo literature as well, along with the tendency to not distinguish between whole and processed carbohydrates.

Putting aside for a moment the question about whether humans evolved to eat these foods back in the Stone Age, it seems nonsensical to ignore the wealth of evidence about how well these foods serve the health and longevity of modern humans. Remember, whole grains are correlated with a reduced risk of death from all causes,[3] and starchy vegetables have

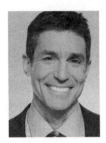

WHOLE FOODIE HERO
David Katz, MD

"The notion that no two nutrition experts agree is, simply, false. The notion that expert opinion in nutrition changes constantly is equally false. It evolves, of course, as science requires; but the truly good advice to eat foods close to nature, consume more plants, and avoid excesses of added sugar or manufacturing mischief in general goes back decades."

Contributions: Katz is a consistent voice of clarity and sanity in the nutritional world and has dedicated himself to cutting through the appearance of confusion and highlighting the clear global evidence-based consensus on what constitutes a healthy diet. To this end he founded the True Health Initiative.

Fun facts: Vivek Murthy, the nineteenth surgeon general of the United States, is a former student of Katz's at Yale and lists Katz as one of his mentors.

Read this: *Disease-Proof: The Remarkable Truth about What Makes Us Well*

Learn more: TrueHealthInitiative.org

played a starring role in the diets of many civilizations. As for legumes, one recent study identified them as "the most important dietary predictor of survival in older people of different ethnicities,"[4] and the daily consumption of these protein- and fiber-packed foods was one of the most significant common denominators among the Blue Zones. In 2007 the American Institute for Cancer Research conducted the most comprehensive analysis of diet and cancer ever performed, and concluded that we should eat whole grains and/or legumes *with every meal.*[5] Paleo's strange demonization of beans and other legumes is the biggest head-scratcher of all from a health perspective.

Ask a Paleo proponent to justify this prohibition on the grounds of health, and he or she will likely say that beans and other legumes contain "antinutrients"—including phytic acid or phytate, which can reduce micronutrient absorption, and lectins, which have been shown in animal studies to impair growth, damage the small intestine, interfere with the pancreas, and destroy skeletal muscle. However, while this sounds ominous, the argument doesn't really hold up under closer scrutiny. Soaking beans overnight and discarding the water before cooking takes care of these issues, as does cooking lentils.

From a health standpoint, then, Paleo diets score high for their focus on real foods instead of processed foods, the embrace of fruits and vegetables, and the caution over dairy, but they overemphasize meat and other animal foods and unnecessarily eliminate healthy whole grains, starchy vegetables, and legumes. If you feel drawn to this dietary philosophy but want to avoid its downsides, we'll offer recommendations for a Whole Foodie variation on the Paleo diet in a moment. First, let's take a closer look at some of the thinking behind this sometimes positive yet sometimes puzzling dietary trend.

Evolution and the "Natural" Human Diet

Looking back into the evolutionary past can certainly provide valuable data in the quest to find the optimum diet for our present and future. However, the idea that a particular slice of that past holds the secret to the "natural" diet is questionable. Different historical times may have produced different climates, environmental challenges, or selection pressures that pushed diets in different directions. Historically, the human diet has been one of change, adaption, and survival—not optimization. We are a constant work in progress, evolutionarily speaking, and it's a mistake to think that some particular point in human or hominid history represents a moment of perfect adaptation to our environment or maximum evolutionary fitness. As evolutionary biologist Marlene Zuk writes in her well-argued book *Paleofantasy: What Evolution Really Tells Us about Sex, Diet, and How We Live,* "The notion that humans got to a point in evolutionary history when their bodies were somehow in sync with the environment, and that sometime later we went astray from those roots—whether because of the advent of agriculture, the invention of the bow and arrow, or the availability of the hamburger—reflects a misunderstanding of evolution."[6]

Zuk suggests that rather than arbitrarily choosing one period, we need to look at the overall thirty million years of primate history. The three million years of the Paleolithic era is only a brief period compared with the long journey of our primate past. Some speculate that if there were a "natural" diet, it would be closer to the leaves, seeds, flowers, nuts, and fruits consumed for much of the twenty million years of hominid development. Another argument can be made that we would find the "natural" diet in the example of our closest genetic cousins, the chimpanzees, bonobos, and gorillas, who eat diets that are between 95% and 100% plant foods.

Even if it were true that the Paleolithic era is in fact the dietary gold mine that adherents like to think, there are respected researchers who take issue with the popular Paleo conclusions about what constituted the diet of the time. For starters, as archaeological geneticist Christina Warinner, PhD, says, "There is no one Paleo diet. There are many, many Paleo diets." Coastal dwellers may have eaten more fish; northern hunter-gatherers in more extreme climates likely ate more meat and animal fats; temperate inhabitants surely ate more fresh fruits and vegetables, and so on. "When we speak about Paleolithic diets," Warinner emphasizes, "it's very important to speak of them in the plural."[7]

Researchers have also questioned another central tenet of Paleo: the predominance of meat. No doubt our ancestors did eat meat when they could hunt and kill it, but it seems unlikely that they ever relied on it to the degree that modern Paleo dieters do. As some have suggested, perhaps the label *hunter-gatherers* should be turned around—*gatherer-hunters* would be more accurate. Yes, prehistoric man gets some of the glory for occasionally bringing down big game, but prehistoric woman was most likely the more important food provider, gathering fruits, seeds, nuts, vegetables, tubers, and all kinds of prehistoric plant foods that played the more important role in the everyday Paleolithic diet.

Anthropologist Nathaniel J. Dominy is one of many researchers and anthropologists who poke holes in the idea that hunted meat played such a central role in Stone Age diets. His research has focused around a particular gene that helps code for amylase, a protein in saliva that breaks down starches into glucose. Other primates besides humans don't have this gene, and it makes Dominy suspect that it is part of what allowed us to take the extraordinary evolutionary leap forward known as the "brain's big bang" and make the journey from our hominid past to *Homo sapiens sapiens* (something Paleo theorists tend to attribute to an increase in meat consumption). After all, Dominy argues, our brain's preferred fuel is glucose. He suggests that humans are not really carnivores but "starchivores," relying on starches to obtain the necessary nutrients for their developing brains: "I would say a mixture of plant foods with a large amount of starch coming from tubers and seeds—that's the fundamental component of the human diet."[8]

This, of course, calls into question another central tenet of the Paleo philosophy—the rejection of starches. Evolutionary biologist Karen Hardy has also argued that starchy vegetables and tubers like yams, squashes, and potatoes played a critical role in the development of the bigger brains that distinguish humans from their predecessors. "The regular consumption of starchy plant foods offers a coherent explanation for the provision of energy to the developing brain during the Late Pliocene and Early Pleistocene," she writes. This idea is backed up by recent evidence that cooking began much earlier than previously believed—as far back as 1.8 million years ago.[9] Other researchers have argued that even grains like wheat and barley played a key role in the human diet long before they were farmed. Evidence has also been found that Neanderthals ate wild varieties of peas and fava beans, contradicting the Paleo claims about legumes.[10] In general, there is plenty of evidence that hominids evolved a largely plant-based eating style, with some animal foods being supplemental, though the proportions over hundreds of thousands of years were probably varied and oft-changing.

It's important to remember that for most of our history, getting enough calories was the primary preoccupation. Even one of the originators of

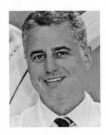

WHOLE FOODIE HERO
Garth Davis, MD

"For doctors to fail to inform patients of the gentlest, safest, most beneficial action they can take to promote their health is nothing short of criminal negligence."

Contributions: Davis is a bariatric (weight-loss) surgeon who has spent considerable time at the heart of America's obesity epidemic. His 2015 book *Proteinaholic* is a carefully researched and passionate refutation of America's obsession with animal protein.

Fun facts: In addition to treating patients at his clinic in Houston, Dr. Davis is also a triathlete who competes around the country while eating a plant-based diet.

Read this: *Proteinaholic: How Our Obsession with Meat Is Killing Us and What We Can Do about It*

Learn more: proteinaholic.com

Paleo, Melvin Konner, acknowledged in a 2016 article that rather than being extreme carnivores, both Neanderthals and early humans were "diet opportunists." In other words, they ate whatever they could get their hands on in order to stay alive. But merely because we *can* and once *did* eat something to survive does not mean we *should* eat tons of it today if we want to thrive. Interestingly, in that same article, Konner distanced himself from contemporary iterations of the diet, comparing his errant creation to Frankenstein's monster.[11]

Konner also backtracked on the argument, advanced in his and Eaton's original paper and repeated by Cordain and others, that the last ten thousand years since the birth of agriculture have not been enough time for our bodies to adapt to digest the more recent foods in our contemporary diets. Science has moved forward since then, and he acknowledges that "in 1985 scientists believed that few genetic changes had occurred since we were all hunting and gathering, say 10,000 years ago. Now we know that lots of genes have changed."[12]

These are just a sampling of the many cogent critiques of Paleo's science. Even if all of these were to be dismissed, the Paleo reading of history turned out to be true, and adherents' conclusions about its significance were borne out, there is still one major problem with the modern Paleo diet: However much we might want to eat like cavemen and cavewomen, we can't.

Let's imagine, for a moment, that we were to take the Paleo philosophy to its extreme and hunt our own meats—they would bear very little resemblance to the lean, wild venison or boar our ancestors would have eaten. The same is true of fruits and vegetables—the ones we eat today have been vastly altered from their wild precursors. In truth, almost all the foods we consume have been transformed over the course of history, and few if any resemble what might have been eaten in the Paleolithic era. Furthermore, modern Paleo dieters seem to overlook the fact that the range of foods available to them from all corners of the world is a far cry from the localized menu of any nomadic hunter-gatherer.

If You're a Whole Foodie...and Paleo

Despite the questionable evolutionary claims made by Paleo advocates, let's not forget the positive principles that their diet continues to promote. Cutting out processed food can only be good. Eating lots of fruits and vegetables and some nuts will extend our lives and protect against disease. Some lean meats and fish can be part of a healthy diet. When seen in this way, the Paleo diet is, as Yale's David Katz writes, "eminently reasonable, and no doubt a vast improvement over the typical American diet." However, he cautions, "When the Paleo Diet label is used to justify a diet of sausages and bacon cheeseburgers, the concept has wandered well off the reservation."[13]

If the Paleo ethos appeals to you, we'd suggest a few adaptions that will make it fit the Whole Foodie philosophy—which might also make it more accurate to the historical diet of our ancestors. Eat lots of fresh vegetables and fruits, and let them fill up the majority of your plate. It's fine to eat some lean meat, fish, and eggs, but keep these to 10% or less of total calories. If you choose to shun grains, at least consider eating starchy root vegetables like yams, squash, sweet potatoes, pumpkin, and potatoes. In place of some meat, make space on your plate for beans and other legumes, as it seems the cavemen probably did too.

Do Humans Need to Eat Animal Foods?

Clearly we don't agree with the Paleo conviction that human beings need large quantities of animal protein to survive and thrive. But do we need any at all? Or would we be better off eating 100% plants?

Throughout these pages we have been recommending a 90+% plant-based diet, which means up to 10% of calories can come from animal foods—meat, fish, dairy products, eggs, and so on. We do this not as a concession or a compromise, but because we feel that the evidence, *from a health perspective*, does not clearly show that a 100% plant-based (or vegan) diet is a better choice. Yes, there are studies showing that people on a vegan or vegetarian diet fare far better than people on the Standard American Diet, with its emphasis on highly processed foods and animal foods. We know that heavy animal product consumption is associated with higher rates of mortality.[14] And, as we shared in chapters 5 and 6, diets with little or no animal products have been shown to reverse heart disease and diabetes. But no study has yet compared people who eat a 100% plant-based whole foods diet with those who include up to 10% animal products. We would love to see such a study conducted.

In today's world, unlike cavemen, most of us do not eat to simply survive. We have the luxury of considering many factors as we choose what to eat, with health being only one of them. We can choose, for ethical reasons, to eat 100% plant-based foods, and by eating skillfully we can do so without compromising health, particularly if we avoid highly processed foods. Once again, we as authors have all made this choice, but we try not to let our ethical convictions cloud our objectivity when it comes to what the science shows.

One question we asked ourselves, when considering whether to recommend a 90+% plant-based or 100% plant-based diet, from a health perspective, is this: Why are there no examples in the historical record of a tribe, culture, or civilization who ate 100% plant-based foods? Once again, it seems highly probable that a *mostly* plant-based omnivorous diet is the one humans have evolved eating and is the one we are best adapted to biologically, and we know that our nearest primate genetic cousins, the chimpanzees and bonobos, are approximately 95% plant-based eaters. Of course history is only a guide, and the fact that neither our evolutionary nor our cultural past includes veganism does not constitute the final word on the optimum diet today.

Among the Blue Zones—the areas in the world where people live the longest, healthiest lives (see chapter 4)—only a small subset of one community (the Loma Linda Adventists) was considered vegan. In the Adventist Health Studies, those who included small amounts of animal products in their diets all had similar health outcomes. All other Blue Zone populations got some percentage of their calories from animal foods—generally a small percentage (10% on average, according to Buettner's meta-analysis).

The best nutritional arguments in favor of the 100% plant-based diet come from those who have successfully used such diets to reverse heart disease and diabetes. Dr. Esselstyn's heart disease prevention program removed all animal products from patients' diets (although he initially allowed some low-fat dairy), as did Dr. Barnard's diabetes reversal diet, while Dr. Ornish's program allowed only egg whites and nonfat dairy in small amounts. The results are compelling, and if you are trying to reverse heart disease or diabetes, you may well want to consider adopting a similar diet.

However, despite the fact that these diets are effective at reversing disease, their long-term health impacts over decades remain to be seen. Veganism is a new dietary approach (the term was invented only in 1944; the practice entered the counterculture in the 1960s and '70s and has become mainstream only in the past couple of decades) and we haven't yet had time to study its long-term effects.

Today's growing vegan movement is a grand experiment, with millions of people eating a diet that is unprecedented in human history. We can measure its positive results on the welfare of animals, on greater environmental sustainability, and on short-term disease reversal, but from the perspective of long-term health, the jury is still out on whether it is superior. Therefore, based on our best reading of the evidence available, we recommend a whole foods, 90+% plant-based diet. To more skillfully optimize your health potential, we recommend that you make the Essential Eight whole food groups part of your regular diet (see chapter 10) as well as consider our supplementation recommendations (see page 174).

Evolution Continues

"We are Stone Agers living in the Space Age," Cordain once claimed. There is truth in this perspective, but falsehood as well. No doubt most of our physiology and instincts were fashioned in the distant past. But we are not cavemen. Cavemen didn't build civilizations or develop complex cultures, nor did they study nutrition with the lens of science. We are part Stone Age *and* part Space Age. Evolution connects us to our distant past and it points us toward our fast-approaching future.

Ultimately, we must deal with life conditions of our own time. We can learn from our past, but we cannot go back. We will never be Paleo again. History moves in one direction. At its best the Paleo movement has taken up the honorable fight to combat the problems of our modern industrialized processed food system, and return to putting real, whole foods on our plates. At its worst it has simply demonized healthy food choices in the name of an imagined past.

With the possible exception of a few historical cultures, many of them born of geographical necessity, humanity has never consumed the degree of animal foods that we currently do in the developed world. Paleo, for all its strengths, has changed nothing about that questionable health experiment, and, in fact, has given it ideological cover. It places the blame for chronic diseases on a series of scapegoat foods and perpetuates America's ongoing fascination with high-protein diets and overreliance on meats. Meanwhile, as we've seen, all the healthiest and longest-lived peoples in the world consume animal foods in limited amounts. It is our conviction that we will not fully address America's chronic disease nightmare, nor reach our true health potential, until both the tenets of the Whole Foods Diet are practiced: eating whole foods *and* eating mostly plants.

A whole foods, largely plant-based diet is the optimum diet today, and it is also the likely diet, when it was possible, of our hunter-gatherer ancestors. A typical person living in Paleolithic times might have enjoyed an occasional fish, or hunted down a deer or even bigger game, but his day-to-day food choices would likely have been a variety of different plants—and lots of them!

One area in which we have a significant advantage over cavemen is in our ability to consciously reflect on, reimagine, and reinvent our diet. We are not confined to the overwhelming necessities of immediate survival, and we have the evolutionary privilege of being able to carefully examine our relationship to our food and choose the best path forward. Our Space Age cognition has some degree of freedom from Stone Age instincts. For example, we may crave fat, salt, and sugar, but we do not need to gorge on hamburgers, fries, and milkshakes all day long. We can recognize our biological predilections, work with our instincts, choose better foods, and even rewire our taste buds (as we will explore in chapter 11). It's important to remember that just because we are drawn to certain foods doesn't mean they are the foods we *should* be eating.

The future is coming fast. Our diets will likely change, and our methods of producing food may change as well—hopefully for the better. The best we can do is learn from the missteps of the twentieth century and not let our food systems get ahead of clearheaded science and good nutrition. There is much we still don't understand about food, but we have more than enough knowledge to live happily and healthily—for a much longer time than our Paleolithic ancestors could have dreamed of.

A Whole Foodie does his or her best to integrate the Stone Age, the Space Age, and our own age. We can learn from the past without romanticizing it, integrate the best of the present without falling prey to its pathologies, and look toward a technologically enhanced future without adopting it blindly. We can follow the best evidence where we have it, and make informed and reasonable decisions where we do not. We can recognize the strengths of approaches like Paleo while not falling prey to its idiosyncratic ideology.

We can, in other words, evolve.

◢ WHOLE FOODIE TAKEAWAYS ◣

• **The upside of the Paleo diet is the emphasis on real food**—along with the encouragement to eat fruits and vegetables and reduce dairy consumption.

• **The downside of the Paleo diet is the overemphasis on meat**—While you don't have to go vegan on the Whole Foods Diet, we do recommend keeping animal foods to 10% or less to avoid the negative health outcomes consistently associated with meat-heavy diets.

• **There is no convincing reason, evolutionary or otherwise, to avoid beans and whole grains**—they are some of the healthiest foods on the planet.

PART II

THE WHOLE FOODIE LIFESTYLE

CHAPTER 9

So, What Should I Eat?

Navigating Everyday Food Choices

"To eat is a necessity, but to eat intelligently is an art."

—*François de La Rochefoucauld*

Black bean and avocado soft corn tacos. Blueberry pancakes. Baked potatoes with mushroom gravy.

Does any of that sound good to you? These are the kinds of delicious, nutritious meals you get to eat on the Whole Foods Diet. If you've read this far, we hope you're thinking seriously about the relationship between your diet and your health, and getting inspired by your own health potential. And you're probably starting to ask the all-important question: *So, what should I eat?*

Our intention in this book is not to dictate what you can or cannot eat—those are decisions only you can make for yourself, informed by the science available, based on your goals, your preferences, and your particular circumstances. While having someone else tell you what to put in your mouth may work for a short-term diet program, we don't believe it's sustainable as a lifestyle. Besides, human beings are contrary creatures and we tend to rebel against the dictates of others. As Dr. Dean Ornish likes to point out, "as soon as I tell somebody what to do, they want to do the opposite...This goes back to the first dietary intervention, when God said, 'Don't eat the apple.'"[1]

To change the way you eat for the long haul, you need to decide how dramatic you want the changes to be and then you need to feel empowered to make those changes. What we intend to do is support you in making those decisions—give you knowledge, tools, and confidence to take your health into your own hands. We hope that what you've read so far has inspired you to *want* to do so—not because we told you that you should, but because you recognize the incredible benefits of making the shift. Above all, we want to make it simple for you to do so—to offer commonsense guidelines that can lift the fog of confusion that too often surrounds healthy eating. In the chapters ahead, you'll find:

- Practical guidance for choosing foods that fit within the Whole Foods Diet
- A list of the Essential Eight food groups that will help optimize the nutritional benefits from your diet
- Insight and guidance to deal with the psychological challenge of changing your habits and evolving your palate
- Helpful tips for dealing with everyday situations

Our recommendations reflect what we conclude is the optimal diet, based on the best science available to us. Do you have to follow these recommendations "perfectly" to see any benefits? We like to look at it this way: every step you take in this direction will directly affect your health, but the more you change, the greater will be the transformation. Do you want to reach and maintain your ideal weight? Get off your medications? Reverse chronic disease? Add years to your life? We think it's important that you know what's optimal and to set your goals high. Too many dietary experts take a patronizing attitude—toning down what science shows is optimal in order to make it more acceptable. We believe you should know what the optimal diet is and then make up your own mind about what you want to do with it.

Once again, the optimal human diet for health and longevity is 100% whole foods, 90+% plant-based. Eat lots of fruits, vegetables, whole grains, and legumes, plus some nuts and seeds. Cut out the highly processed foods, especially refined flours, sugars, and oils. And if you choose to eat animal foods, keep them to less than 10% of your calories. We as authors each strive to eat this way, and we're motivated to do so by how healthy, vital, and nourished we feel every day.

Of course, there are occasional circumstances when it's just not possible to make the optimal choice, and then we choose the best that is available. And there are times when we choose to enjoy something we would not consider to be the healthiest food—but these are rare exceptions, not the rule. Don't let perfectionism trip you up. If you listen to people in the plant-based eating movement, you'll probably hear terms like "plant-perfect" and "plant-pure." While well intentioned, in our experience such language can be counterproductive, leading people to aim for a perfection that, for them, may be impossible to achieve. That's not to say there's anything wrong with striving to be the best you can be, but the downside of trying to be perfect is that any small slip is perceived as failure, leading too easily into a negative spiral of self-blame and doubt. And when we feel bad about ourselves, it's all too easy to seek comfort in our old habits. We feel we've failed anyway, so why even try?

Instead, own your choices and make better ones the next day. Learn from your mistakes and try again—things are often easier the second time around. Challenge yourself to go a little further than you think is possible, then let the results you experience inspire you to go even further.

When it comes to diet, what matters most is the overall pattern. Get the big pieces in place: *100% whole foods, 90+% plant based*. Dr. Pam Popper, nutritionist, health educator, and founder of Wellness Forum Health, compares a dietary pattern to a combination lock, with the numbers representing the major elements of the diet. All the numbers need to line up for it to open—it's not enough to get just some of them right.[2] If you shift to a primarily plant-based diet but keep eating large quantities of highly processed foods, you won't see the benefits. And if you choose to eat whole foods, but continue to get a large percentage of calories from animal products, the same holds.

Our advice to you is to focus on unlocking your health potential by establishing the overall pattern. Within this pattern there is plenty of room for variation based on preference, health, life circumstances, and so on. On a day-to-day basis, make food choices consciously, knowing that the closer you keep to that optimal diet, the better chance you'll have for optimal health.

So what are "better" choices? Food does not fall into two simple categories labeled "good" and "bad." It's more accurate to think of it as a continuum, with the most health-promoting foods on one end and the most disease-promoting foods on the other. Between those two extremes lie many of the foods that the average person encounters every day. In order to decide which of them you want, let's return to the two general rules introduced in chapter 1. These two rules can act as your compass for the choices you make every day.

A Whole Foodie…
eats whole foods instead of highly processed foods
and
eats mostly plant foods (90+% of calories).

Follow these two rules and fairly quickly you may notice more energy and vitality. Continue eating this way, and you'll naturally reach your optimum weight and find that many health complaints resolve themselves. Let's take a closer look at how each of these rules plays out in specific situations.

Eating Whole Foods Instead of Highly Processed Foods

Processing—it's a simple word that contains a multitude of problems. It can turn a healthy, nutritious food into one that has little nutritional value left and may even make you sick. Let's revisit the key distinctions when it comes to the transformation of food.

Unprocessed or Whole Foods

These are "real foods." These foods are essentially intact, close to the form in which they grew. None of their essential nutritious parts have been removed, and no unhealthy substances (sugar, salt, oil, or chemicals such as artificial flavors, preservatives, or colors) have been added to them. This includes all types of whole fruits and vegetables, whole grains, beans and other legumes, and nuts and seeds, as well as unprocessed animal foods. You'll often find unprocessed foods in the perimeter aisles of grocery stores, as well as at farmers markets. They usually don't need much if any packaging, nor do they feature long ingredient lists. They won't contain preservatives, and many need to be kept in the refrigerator and consumed soon after purchase, unless they've been dried, like beans and whole grains, or purchased frozen.

Whole plant foods are always healthy choices. Eat these foods in abundance, embracing the wonderful variety of nature's bounty—from crunchy green vegetables to hearty, nourishing beans to comforting starchy vegetables to wholesome grains to sweet and vibrant fruits.

The only time we recommend caution in the category of whole plant foods is with calorie-dense varieties like nuts, seeds, olives, avocados, and dried fruits. While these play a part in a healthy diet, they contain a much higher ratio of calories to weight. As we discussed in chapter 2, it can be wise to limit consumption of calorie-dense foods (unless you are someone who needs extra calories, like an endurance athlete) and focus on foods that are rich in nutrients and highly satiating, but lower in calories, especially if you are trying to lose weight.

Minimally Processed Foods

These are a harder category to define, but we use this term to mean that while some processing has occurred, the food is still nutritious and has not been overly adulterated. This includes products that are made from whole foods, like whole grain flours and pastas; whole grain breads and tortillas; certain soy products like tofu and tempeh; nut butters and unsweetened nondairy milks; and so on. Many of these still contain all the parts of the whole food, but it has often been broken down into smaller pieces. Once again, we consider these equivalent to whole foods, following Dr. Michael Greger's definition: "Nothing bad added, nothing good taken away." These foods are healthy choices, compared with more heavily processed options, especially when they are used as a vehicle for eating more whole plant foods. Whole grain pasta primavera, bursting with beautiful spring vegetables, is one example; another is whole corn tacos stuffed with beans, grilled veggies, and fresh salsa.

With any processed food, even minimally processed ones, it's always important to pay attention to what has been taken away and what may have been added. The more fiber that has been removed, the more calorie dense the food is likely to be (see chapter 2). White rice is a bit more calorie dense

Tips for Reading Food Labels

If you focus on unprocessed, whole natural foods, most of them won't even have labels to read. When you do buy something that comes in a package, it's important to read the nutrition label (the one on the back) and make sure that you:

• **Limit added fats**—Keep the "calories from fat" to 20% or less of total calories, and avoid foods high in saturated fat or containing partially hydrogenated oils.

• **Limit added salt**—Look for a 1:1 ratio or less of sodium (milligrams) to calories.

• **Limit added sugars**—Make sure they don't appear in the first five ingredients.

• **Avoid refined grains**—Choose grain products that are 100% whole grain.

Thanks to Jeff Novick, MS, RD, for permission to adapt his label-reading system.

than brown rice for this reason and has had its nutritional value reduced with the removal of the bran layer and germ along with all that beneficial fiber. However, it's not a bad choice if you don't have the option of brown, particularly if it becomes the bed for a big pile of fresh vegetables and beans. In general, when buying packaged foods and breads, we try to choose those with at least one to two grams of fiber per fifty calories—so if you look at a food label and it has one hundred calories per serving, ideally it should have at least two to four grams of fiber per serving.

With minimally processed foods, it's always important to read the ingredients closely. Too much added salt, oil, or sugar can turn a simple plant-based food into a health risk. Don't be fooled by health claims on the packaging. A whole grain, vegan, gluten-free doughnut is still a doughnut, and contains plenty of sugar and oil. Always look for products with the fewest added ingredients.

For example, if you buy almond milk, choose the unsweetened version without added oil or salt, or if you feel ambitious, you can make it at home (see technique, page 266). When you choose bread, make sure it's 100% whole grain. For condiments, sauces, or spreads, pay attention to added sugar, oil, or salt per calorie. If it has a list of ten or twenty ingredients, and half the terms are in science-speak, you can be fairly certain it's not a real food.

Many people might consider freshly squeezed fruit and vegetable juices minimally processed plant foods—after all, they've only gone through a juicer. However, the transformation those fruits and vegetables have undergone is significant. While they retain many of their nutrients, they have lost all of their essential fiber, along with some nutrients bound to that fiber. Therefore, they deliver a concentrated dose of sugars without the natural fiber that helps you metabolize them. As Dr. Garth Davis writes, "It turns out fruits and vegetables are perfectly packaged. The sugars in fruit are designed to work almost like a time-release pill, due to their relationship and binding with the fiber. When you juice, you uncouple this perfect package by removing the fiber." He adds that in this light, the idea of a prolonged juice fast for detoxification makes little sense, given that "fiber is the most detoxifying substance we can consume. It literally scrubs your insides. You can't detox without fiber."[3] Rather than drink a juice, consider blending fruits and vegetables into a smoothie (see page 267 for our favorite smoothie recipes), or, better still, eat them whole.

Highly Processed or Ultraprocessed Foods

These foods have been significantly altered from their original form, often to the point that they bear no resemblance to something that grew out of the ground or on a tree. Stripped of fiber and other essential parts and often packed with added salt, fat, sugar, and chemicals, they become calorie rich and nutrient poor. This category includes all refined grains and products made from them, such as white flour, white pasta, cookies, and so on. Oils and margarines also fall into this category (see page 170), as do candy, sweets, and anything that's been deep-fried, such as tortilla chips and French fries.

These foods tend to have long ingredient lists full of unrecognizable terms, and they often make all kinds of health claims on the packaging. "Added Calcium!" "Heart Healthy!" "Fiber Rich!" You've probably seen such claims on breakfast cereals, bags of chips, granola bars, and many other products. Michael

The Perils of Processing

Here's a reminder of three essentials you need to understand about processing:

Processing removes or breaks down fiber. When fiber is broken down or removed, many important benefits of fiber are lost. (see page 69).

Processing concentrates calories. Because fiber has been removed or broken down and water has been removed, processed foods pack more calories into less bulk, meaning that to feel satisfied, you're likely to eat more calories than your body needs.

Processing adds unhealthy substances. Too often, as food is processed, it gets loaded with oils, sugars, salt, and chemicals, increasing its calorie count and other health risks without any nutritional benefit.

Pollan points out, that in contrast, the food that is unquestionably good for you—fresh fruits and vegetables—often doesn't have the political clout or the advertising dollars to tout its benefits. "Don't take the silence of the yams as a sign that they have nothing valuable to say about health,"[4] he cautions.

Whatever the packaging claims, most highly processed foods have little or no nutritional benefit; in fact, they often have adverse effects on health. They do not have any place in an optimal human diet.

The chart on page 165 shows what happens to some common foods as they move through the spectrum of processing—starting out as wholesome, nutrient-rich foods and ending up as calorie-dense, nutrient-poor shadows of themselves. The Whole Foods Diet focuses on the left-hand side of this spectrum.

Eating Mostly Plant Foods (90+% of Calories)

While the distinction between whole and processed foods is a continuum, the distinction between plant foods and animal foods is a clear line. If it grew out

The Continuum of Processing

- *Wheat berry → Cracked wheat → Whole wheat flour → White flour → Cookie*
- *Soybean → Tempeh → Soy milk → Soy isolate → Soy hot dog*
- *Strawberry → Dried strawberry → Strawberry jelly → Strawberry ice cream*
- *Orange → Orange juice → Orange sorbet → Orange soda*

of the ground, on a tree, or on a vine, it's a plant. If it had a face, or a mother, or came from something that had a face or a mother, it's an animal food.

Some people, for ethical reasons, may choose not to eat any animal products, or only to eat dairy products and eggs. Putting aside the ethical issues for now, from a health perspective, our recommendation is that plants should make up *at least 90%* of your overall calorie intake.

If the term *calorie* reminds you of many failed attempts at "calorie-counting" diets, let us clarify that with a whole foods, plant-based diet you don't need to obsess over calories. If the majority of meals come from a variety of whole plant foods, you'll naturally satisfy your nutritional needs and appetite without overeating (see chapter 2). However, when it comes to animal foods, we think it's worth taking a calorie-focused approach, simply because most of us are accustomed to overeating these foods. You may need to do a little calorie calculation at first until you get used to the appropriate portions.

Based on a two-thousand-calorie-per-day diet, the box on page 167 shows some examples how that 10% or less might look. You may need to adjust for your particular caloric needs—you can easily find tools online to calculate your daily average (we like the website Cronometer.com, which offers many other helpful free tools as well). You might take a "condiment" approach, in which you use animal foods not as the centerpiece of your meal but as a topping or enhancement, as is common in traditional Asian cooking.

Alternately, if you love to enjoy a larger serving of your favorite animal foods, think of them as occasional treats once or twice a week at most, or save them for celebratory occasions, as many of the world's longest-lived cultures do. This strategy means you'll eat your maximum

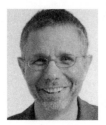

WHOLE FOODIE HERO
Jeff Novick, MS, RDN

"We aren't healthy (or unhealthy) because of any one food, good or bad. What makes us healthy or unhealthy are our overall dietary and lifestyle patterns."

Contributions: With his unparalleled nutritional expertise, Novick has been a powerful advocate of plant-based eating for decades, contributing to many important health initiatives. Known as an accomplished teacher, he has helped develop educational material for the McDougall Program, Engine 2, Whole Foods Market, the Pritikin Longevity Center, and others.

Fun facts: A former French pastry chef, Novick has many talents and even worked as a salesman for Kraft Foods, selling cheese. He is not only an expert in nutrition, but in meditation, which he has been practicing for more than thirty years.

Watch this: "Calorie Density: How to Eat More, Weigh Less, and Live Longer" (available for free on YouTube)

Learn more: JeffNovick.com

of 10% animal foods in one or two meals for the entire week.

If you choose to eat animal foods, be aware how the animals are raised. Modern industrial factory farming has made animal foods widely available and affordable, but at significant cost—both to the well-being of animals and to your health. From a health perspective, common practices that are cause for concern include treating livestock with antibiotics and growth hormones, and feeding them corn and other products that are far removed from their natural diet. While people in all the Blue Zones ate small amounts of animal foods, none of them ate modern factory-farmed versions. We recommend, if you choose to eat animal foods, that you follow these guidelines:

- *Choose grass-fed, organic, antibiotic-free meat and dairy products, and pasture-raised chickens and eggs.*
- *Choose wild-caught fish and seafood where possible, and avoid those more likely to contain toxins such as mercury*—Species to avoid tend to be those that are longer lived and higher up on the food chain, including tuna, swordfish, and king mackerel.
- *Avoid processed meats.* The World Health Organization recently categorized processed meats as a Group 1 carcinogen, alongside cigarettes and asbestos.[5] If you decide to eat meat, choose unprocessed forms and stay away from hot dogs, salami, bologna, bacon, ham, and the like.

Food Choice FAQs

We hope you're starting to feel confident about making important distinctions that will make all the difference for your health and well-being. But you probably still have questions. Let's try to answer a few of them.

Animal Foods as Condiments

Once a day you could add just one of these foods to your salad or stir-fry, or include it as a side dish. That would put you at your ≤10% daily limit on animal foods. If you're aiming for closer to 5%, do this every other day.

Grilled salmon (four ounces)
Grilled chicken breast (four ounces)
Broiled steak (four ounces)
Shrimp (six ounces)
Goat cheese (two ounces)

Note that with all these examples, we recommend choosing cooking methods that don't involve added oil—which immediately adds extra calories you don't need, along with other health risks. (See page 271 for more tips on cooking without oil.)

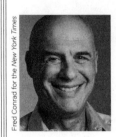

Fred Conrad for the New York Times

WHOLE FOODIE HERO
Mark Bittman

"The truly healthy alternative to that chip is not a fake chip; it's a carrot."

Contributions: As a high-profile *New York Times* columnist and prolific cookbook author, Bittman has been an influential and educational voice for improving America's food culture and a promoter of real food with an emphasis on plants.

Fun facts: Bittman created the VB6 ("vegan before six") movement, encouraging people to eat only plants until their evening meal as a means to better health and weight loss.

Read this: *A Bone to Pick*

Learn more: MarkBittman.com

Where Will I Get My Protein?

Human beings need protein to survive and thrive. Protein has become associated in the American mind with energy, vitality, and strength—like an all-purpose wonder nutrient. Feeling a bit low? Getting a bit skinny? Looking a bit pale? You must not be getting enough protein. And many people fear that if you eat a plant-based diet, you definitely will lack this critical macronutrient. "Where do you get your protein?" is the common refrain, since most people associate protein almost entirely with animal foods, and are convinced we need a lot of it. Both of these assumptions are unfounded.

First, plants contain protein. After all, how do you think the elephants and giraffes live off of them? Beans and other legumes, whole grains, seeds, nuts, and even green vegetables are all wonderful sources of protein. And not only do plants contain protein, they may be a healthier source of it. Using data from the Nurses' Health Study, researchers at Harvard School of Public Health analyzed the diets of more than 130,000 people, and found that greater consumption of protein from animal sources, especially red and processed meats, increased risk of mortality. Alternatively, the researchers found that greater consumption of

The Whole Foods Diet at a Glance

Foods to Eat Freely

Vegetables, fruits, intact whole grains and whole grain pasta, beans and other legumes, starchy vegetables

Foods to Eat in Moderation*

Whole grain breads, tortillas, crackers, dry cereals, tofu, tempeh, soy and nut milks, nuts, seeds, avocados, olives, dried fruit

Especially if you're trying to lose weight

Meat (unprocessed), fish, eggs, and dairy products (keep animal foods to 10% or less of your caloric intake)

Foods to Avoid

Refined flours, sugar, oils, baked goods, sweets, junk food, soda

Lunch meats, bacon, sausages, hot dogs, salami

---

plant-based protein was associated with a longer life.[6] Perhaps this is because most meat, which is a common source of protein, is also a significant source of extra calories, fat, and other problematic nutrients—especially when consumed in the amounts common in American diets today. The healthiest diets we know of that include meat do so only in limited amounts.

Second, Americans tend to vastly overestimate the amount of protein needed. We drink protein shakes, eat protein bars, go on high-protein diets, and choose breakfast cereals that advertise protein content. Yet, as a nation, we are far from protein deficient. Most people who worry about not getting enough protein—and who always look for more—are not aware of how much they already get nor how much they need for optimum health. Government recommendations are forty-six grams of protein per day for the average woman and fifty-six grams of protein per day for the average man,[7] but the average American woman aged twenty to forty-nine gets more than seventy, and the average man age twenty to forty-nine gets well over one hundred.[8] We may in fact get too much protein, which is not necessarily a good thing. Excess protein can stress systems and make kidneys and liver work too hard, among other things.

It's virtually impossible to be protein deficient if you eat enough whole food calories. Yes, that's right. If you eat enough whole foods (even just plant foods), you don't need to worry about protein. So the concern about getting enough protein on a plant-based diet is unfounded. Yet, as Dr. Garth Davis writes, "Despite decades of evidence…the presupposition that protein is good and more is better is still firmly implanted in our mind."[9] Davis, whose 2015 book *Proteinaholic* dismantles that presupposition beyond any reasonable doubt, likens the American attitude to this nutrient to an addiction. "Our obsessive and mindless overconsumption of protein fits the pattern of addiction, and its health consequences—for individuals and society as a whole—are no less serious in the long term."[10]

We promise you that a whole foods, plant-based diet will not be protein deficient. Plant sources of protein are perfectly adequate. Forget the common myth that while meat is a complete source of protein, rice and beans need to be combined to deliver all the essential amino acids. It doesn't work like that. Rice or beans, like almost any other whole plant food, are complete in and of themselves. (Check for yourself on any nutrition calculator[11]).Eating lots of whole plant foods not only provides enough protein, it also protects from getting too much, which should be your bigger concern.

Why Are Oils Off-Limits?

The Whole Foods Diet recommends staying away from all refined, extracted oils. That includes canola oil, olive oil, sunflower oil, corn oil, coconut oil, and anything you find beside them on the shelf. For many Americans, that may come as a surprise. Of all the highly processed foods that we tend to eat daily, vegetable oils are not on most people's list of concerns. We use them for cooking, we douse our salads in them, and these days some people even blend them into their coffee. Many consider certain oils—olive oil and coconut oil in particular—to be health foods, even superfoods. However, there are several problems with oils, starting with them being largely devoid of any nutritional value beyond fat.

Oils are nutrient poor. Olives, corn, coconuts, and sunflower seeds all contain nutrients, in their whole food forms. Olive oil, corn oil, coconut oil, and sunflower oil have been extracted in such a way that removes these beneficial nutrients, along with fiber, leaving only empty calories. As you can see from the chart below, extra virgin olive oil and coconut oil barely contain more nutrients than sugar, yet deliver more than double the calories.

Per 100 calories	Extra Virgin Olive Oil	Coconut Oil	Sugar
Amount	2.5 teaspoons	2.5 teaspoons	6.2 teaspoons
Saturated Fat (% calories)	1.6 grams (14%)	9.2 grams (83%)	0
Fiber	0	0	0
Omega-3 fatty acids	0.1 grams	0	0
Omega-6 fatty acids	1.1 grams	0.2 grams	0
Omega-6 to omega-3 ratio (goal is 2:1–4:1)	11:1	Unable to calculate because no omega-3 fatty acids	0
Vitamins	Small amount of vitamin E and vitamin K	0% RDA	0% RDA
Minerals	Trace amount of iron	0% RDA	0% RDA
Protein	0	0	0
Calorie Density	4,000 calories per pound	3,900 calories per pound	1,750 calories per pound

Thanks to Jeff Novick, MS, RD, for permission to adapt this chart from his work.

Oils are among the most calorie-dense foods on the planet. A single tablespoon of oil contains 120 calories. Because oils contain no fiber, they deliver concentrated energy but no bulk, driving up calorie count without filling the stomach or meeting a nutrient need. Oils, in other words, make it exceedingly easy to overeat—as if we needed any more help. Let's say you were to sit down to dinner, starting with a salad, followed by a whole grain pasta dish with some broccoli on the side. If you choose an oil-free salad dressing (see formula, page 279), serve the pasta in oil-free Marinara Sauce (see recipe, page 283), and steam the broccoli, you have a delicious and satisfying meal that may deliver three or four hundred calories. However, if you drench your salad in an oil-based dressing, pour some olive oil on your pasta, and sauté the broccoli, you could be looking at seven or eight hundred calories—more than a cheeseburger and fries! Set the oil aside, and you'll make staying in shape much easier.

You may have heard that the polyunsaturated fats in oils are better than other types of fats. The reality is that many vegetable oils tend to be high in omega-6 fatty acids, and Americans in general get far too many of those already, especially relative to omega-3 fatty acids (what we really need more of). An extreme imbalance in the ratio between these two (typical American diets can be as high as 15:1) has been implicated in a host of health ills, including cancer, autoimmune and inflammatory diseases, and other chronic conditions.[12] Decreasing vegetable oil can be a quick and virtuous route to improving that critical health ratio (experts suggest in the range of 2:1 to 4:1 is optimal).

Another concern with extracted, polyunsaturated plant oils is that they are susceptible to oxidation, which is implicated in tissue damage, aging, and other health complications.[13] They have also been implicated in cardiovascular disease risks, actually making the plaques in the blood vessels worse.[14]

In general, we don't feel there are good and bad oils; rather, they range from bad to worse. Extracting all the fat from a whole food and putting it in a bottle to consume as oil is no healthier than taking all the carbohydrate from a whole food and putting it in a bag to consume as sugar. For all these reasons, we recommend for optimum health to avoid all oils. This means being aware of foods that have added oils in the ingredient list, steering clear of fried and sautéed foods, and learning to love oil-free salads. See page 279 for an easy way to make oil-free salad dressing and see page 271 for tips on how to cook easily and efficiently without oil. If you want richer flavors associated with oils and fats (in spreads, sauces, dressings, and so on), use whole foods like nuts and seeds, olives, or avocados as whole or blended ingredients (see recipe for Oil-Free Herb Pesto on page 299).

What Sweeteners Should I Choose?

We do not recommend using any extracted or concentrated sweeteners, whether in the form of white table sugar, high-fructose corn syrup, or any of the so-called "natural" sweeteners like maple syrup, honey, agave nectar, and so on. If you're trying to eat a whole foods, plant-based diet, we recommend sticking to fruit to satisfy your sweet tooth. If you want to experiment with whole food desserts, dates make a good sweetener (see recipe for Sweet Potato Chocolate Mousse on page 305).

Can I Use Salt?

There is nothing health promoting about added sodium other than when it helps get whole plant foods into your body. That being the case, we recommend using as little added sodium as necessary. When you use it, aim to add it to your plate rather than cook with it in a recipe; you'll get a better bang for your buck because you can taste more and use less. Over time you will find that you need less salt as you stay mindful of it in your diet and your taste buds evolve.

Can I Drink Alcohol?

You may have read recent headlines claiming a glass of wine is better for you than an hour at the gym, tequila is good for your bones, and alcohol can protect against diabetes. While much is made of studies showing possible benefits of alcoholic drinks, wine in particular, we've yet to see convincing evidence that they should be considered a health food. And we all know the dangers of alcohol—its addictive properties and the role it plays in too many accidents. Plus, there is increasing evidence for a link between alcohol consumption and certain cancers.[15]

However, we also recognize that alcohol has been a part of human culture for millennia, and it plays a key role in bringing people together in convivial settings, as is demonstrated in almost all the Blue Zones (see chapter 4). Whatever choices you make around alcohol, keep in mind that it is also high in calories, and may deter efforts at weight loss.

Is It Important to Choose Organic?

The most important dietary change you can make is to eat more fruits and vegetables. A 90+% plant-based diet is going to be significantly healthier than a Standard American Diet even if you are not always able to eat certified organic produce. However, if you have the option, choosing organic has the added benefit of keeping chemical pesticides out of your food chain. We certainly think this is a wise choice, but it's much less important than the choice to eat more fruits and vegetables. One study estimated that if just half the US population increased fruit and vegetable consumption, approximately 20,000 cancer cases per year could be prevented, while only up to ten cancer cases per year could be caused by the added pesticide consumption.[16]

Where Will I Get My Calcium?

Many Americans have grown up associating calcium exclusively with dairy products, milk in particular. If you're concerned that reducing your animal food intake will lead to calcium deficiency, don't worry. In fact, the body actually absorbs calcium from many plant foods, like kale and broccoli, for instance, more easily than from milk. Even nuts, seeds, and legumes are significant plant sources of calcium that may not be commonly considered.[17]

What Supplements Do I Need?

If you choose to eat a mostly plant-based diet, we encourage you to do so skillfully, with appropriate supplementation. We know that a vegan diet with no supplementation whatsoever may result in lower levels of certain nutrients (compared to nonvegans). For those vegans or near-vegans committed to a healthy whole foods diet, these concerns are largely mitigated, but not entirely erased. So what, if any, supplements should you take?

B12? Yes

The one nutrient that is indisputably lacking in a vegan or mostly plant-based diet is vitamin B12.[18] *We believe that B12 supplementation should be nonnegotiable for pure vegans,*[19] and is also likely to be beneficial for those eating 10% or less of their calories from animal foods.[20]

Zinc, Iodine, Iron, Calcium? No

Many of the nutrients that raise deficiency concerns for vegans can be adequately attained from whole plant foods.[21] This applies to commonly raised questions around nutrients like zinc, iodine, iron, and calcium. In general, supplementation should not be necessary for a skillful Whole Foodie eating a healthy whole foods, plant-based diet.[22] Indeed, most plant foods are rich in a diversity of nutrients, and in general there is little reason to be concerned about inadequate levels. But if you would like to bump up your overall intake of these nutrients, here are some plant foods that are extra rich in these four minerals:

> **Zinc**—Most beans (e.g., adzuki, garbanzo, white), seeds (e.g., pumpkin, sesame, squash), and whole grains (e.g., whole wheat, oats, quinoa), dried mushrooms
> **Iodine**—Sea vegetables (e.g., dulse, kelp)
> **Calcium**—Most leafy green vegetables (e.g., collards, broccoli, arugula) and beans (e.g., adzuki, garbanzo, white)
> **Iron**—Most leafy greens (e.g., collards, broccoli, arugula), legumes (e.g., adzuki, garbanzo, white), and whole grains (e.g., whole wheat, oats, quinoa)

DHA? It's Complicated

Unfortunately, the science supporting supplementation on largely plant-based diets is by no means settled. Many people, including highly reputable doctors and nutritionists, have different perspectives and recommendations vary. This is especially true when it comes to whether to recommend supplementation of EPA/DHA, or long-chain omega-3 fatty acids. The concern is that plant-based diets tend to be lower in these essential fats. The richest natural source of preformed EPA/DHA is fish, especially oily fishes such as wild-caught salmon, mackerel, and tuna, so if you eat a diet that is less than 100% plant based, you can get preformed EPA/DHA by including wild-caught fish or seafood in some meals. However, because of the contamination of many fish with mercury, dioxin, PCBs, and other pollutants, eating too much fish comes with its own risks[23] (and these concerns appear to apply to fish oil supplements as well).[24] Therefore, it is advisable to add other foods containing omega-3s to your diet. Many whole plant foods contain omega-3 fatty acids, and some plant foods are particularly rich in them, including flaxseeds, chia seeds, hemp seeds, walnuts, leafy greens, and soybeans. However, the omega-3 fatty acids in these foods come in a "short-chain" form called ALA, which the body must convert into "long-chain" EPA/DHA. So the question arises: Is it worth supplementing EPA/DHA in order to optimize EPA/DHA levels and long-term health? The authors of this book have come to different conclusions. We will present them separately.

Dr. Matthew Lederman and *Dr. Alona Pulde:* Do those with a plant-based diet benefit from supplementing with preformed EPA/DHA? The answer to this question has yet to be clearly determined. The lower level of DHA in vegan populations has not been conclusively linked to disease or deficiency (unlike with B12, where a link is well established). Moreover, you might be interested to know that a large study of more than fourteen thousand people found that those who didn't eat fish seemed to convert enough ALA to EPA/DHA, bringing them to levels close to those of fish eaters.[25] Still, there is preliminary evidence that some potential benefits to brain health may be associated with supplementation.[26] As a result, some experts believe that it is advisable to supplement EPA/DHA routinely, while others, ourselves included, feel that the current evidence is not robust enough to support recommending supplementation preventatively to the average person.

Our recommendation here is that you look to your diet, your personal history, and your risk-to-benefit profile to make that decision. Some people simply have no significant family history and feel well, and as such may choose to wait for better evidence to come out before routinely supplementing. On the other hand, if you have a strong family history of brain-related disorders, you may be more inclined to measure your omega-3 index[27] and, if it is low,[28] consider supplementation. If you choose to supplement, we recommend an algae-based EPA/DHA supplement free of the environmental contaminants found in fish oil supplements.[29] No matter what supplementation path you choose, you should continue to consume whole plant foods rich in omega-3 fatty acids and take steps that will optimize your ability to convert short- to long-chain forms

MY WHOLE FOODIE STORY

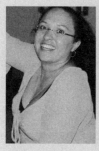 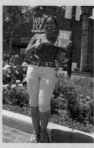

Rebeca Atkins, 46, Fremont, California

There's nothing like almost losing a parent to make one think seriously about getting healthy. Within just a few months of each other, both my parents faced major health crises. My mother had a very bad episode with her Alzheimer's disease, and then my father had an aneurysm and had to have a highly risky brain surgery. Miraculously, he made it through, but all of this made me ask myself how I could avoid these same things happening to me one day. I was thirty pounds overweight and my cholesterol was high.

My first opportunity to make a change came in January 2014, when I did Rip Esselstyn's 28-Day Engine 2 Diet Challenge. My team leader at Whole Foods Market supported several of us through the challenge, making sure we always had the meals available in the break room. That was the first time I experienced the health-transforming impact of plant-based food. My husband joined me, and by the end of the month, I had lost thirteen pounds and he had lost ten. Soon after that I attended Rip's seven-day Immersion in Arizona. I came back home with a new lifestyle and the knowledge I needed to change my future.

Within a year I lost thirty-one pounds and my husband lost thirty. My cholesterol returned to a normal range. I feel that I was given a new beginning. One of my favorite parts of my job today is working with the Whole Kids Foundation to teach kids how to enjoy healthy food. And now, when customers ask me questions about healthy eating, I have the right answers for them, and I am proud to be an example for them to see.

(e.g., minimize alcohol[30] and minimize added oils and other sources of omega-6 fatty acids,[31] which the average person consumes in excess).

John Mackey: I have come to a different conclusion from my colleagues about EPA/DHA supplementation. We need omega-3 essential fatty acids in every cell of our bodies, but EPA/DHA is particularly critical to the development and healthy maintenance of the most important organ in our body—the brain. A large part of the structure of the brain is, in fact, made up of EPA/DHA. The concerns around inadequate levels and brain function are to be taken seriously. Studies have clearly shown that low EPA/DHA levels are associated with slightly lower overall brain volume.[32] While our brain does naturally lose some size as we age, there is evidence that EPA/DHA levels that consistently fall below certain thresholds may exacerbate that natural process. Studies also show that many vegans (and not just vegans but many Americans in general) fall below generally accepted EPA/DHA thresholds. It may eventually prove to be true that a whole foods, plant-based eater will naturally end up converting all the EPA/DHA needed for healthy brain function, and that this is more an issue for less healthy vegan diets and those on Standard American Diets. However, the results of a randomized controlled trial published in 2013 suggest that EPA/DHA supplementation can improve cognitive function and brain health, at least in older adults.[33] So while Matt and Alona are correct in saying that the evidence for long-term deficiency in plant-based diets is not yet conclusive, I feel that prudence, in this instance, falls on the side of action. There is little downside to supplementation, and it may prove beneficial to long-term health and cognitive well-being. In addition to consciously consuming plant foods rich in omega-3s, I support EPA/DHA supplementation and personally take 250 milligrams a day derived from algae (perfectly acceptable for vegans and vegetarians).

CHAPTER 10

The Essential Eight

Health-Promoting Foods to Eat Every Day

"What you include in your diet is as important as what you exclude."

—*Dean Ornish, MD*

When we hear the word *diet*, we tend to associate it with the prohibition of certain foods. However, health isn't just about cutting out the "bad" stuff; it's also about loading up on the "good" stuff—and by good, we mean delicious *and* nutritious!

The variety of nutrient-rich, health-promoting plant foods is endless, and the good news is, they're all good for you! However, different food groups provide different benefits. Nutritional science continues to uncover the secrets of nature's best medicine—food—and every day, it seems, we learn more about the specific compounds in particular fruits and vegetables that promote health. It's a fascinating topic, and although we prefer to focus on whole foods instead of isolated nutrients, it never hurts to learn more about why those whole foods are so powerful at fighting disease and extending life span. To help you become a more skillful eater and maximize the benefits from your diet, we've come up with a list of food groups we call the Essential Eight. When you learn how to prepare these foods in ways that bring out their amazing flavors, you can fill your plate with goodness and leave less and less room for anything else.

How often should you try to eat these foods? As often as you can and ideally every day! While it sometimes might not be possible to eat every

The Essential Eight

1. Whole grains and starchy vegetables
2. Beans and other legumes
3. Berries
4. Other fruits
5. Cruciferous vegetables
6. Leafy greens
7. Nonstarchy vegetables
8. Nuts and seeds

single one, every day, get in the habit of seeing how many you can check off daily, just to keep them in your awareness. We keep this list on the fridge door, or somewhere prominent in the kitchen, as an easy reference.

1. Whole Grains and Starchy Vegetables

One thing many people love about a whole foods, plant-based diet is that it includes the comforting starchy "carb" foods that so many other diets misguidedly tell us to avoid. Sweet and earthy yams, hearty winter squashes, tender juicy corn, and even the much-loved potato, as well as all the varieties of tasty, satisfying whole grains can find a regular place on the Whole Foodie plate. In this category we also include grainlike seeds—such as quinoa, millet, amaranth, buckwheat, and teff—which are nutritionally similar to grains.

Always keep in mind the important and often-missed distinction between whole carbohydrates, like whole grains and starchy vegetables, versus highly processed, refined carbohydrates. While the latter are to be avoided, the former play a key role in an optimum diet. In fact, not only should you be sure to eat whole grains and starchy vegetables, but they also should make up the bulk of your calorie intake.

Carbohydrates are the best energy source humans have available,

What Is an Antioxidant?

If you've been paying attention to dietary trends and nutritional fads over the past few years, you're sure to have heard the term *antioxidant*, usually accompanied by a promise that these miraculous substances will slow the aging process or protect you from disease. Whether antioxidants themselves provide the actual health benefit or they are a marker for other health-promoting nutrients (some of which we may not have even discovered yet) in a particular food, the bottom line is that foods high in antioxidants also tend to be high in health benefits!

Antioxidants are compounds found in certain foods that appear to help fight against the cell-damaging effects of a particular type of unstable molecule called *free radicals*. Antioxidants can safely interact with free radicals and stabilize or neutralize them, preventing damage to cells and organs.

Antioxidants are mostly found in plant foods, including vegetables, fruits, grains, and nuts. Their presence is often signaled by bold, bright color—another good reason to "eat the rainbow," as nutritionists say. A recent study measuring the antioxidant content of more than 3,100 foods found that plant foods were on average sixty-four times more antioxidant rich than animal foods, and concluded that herbs and spices, followed by berries, are the most antioxidant-rich foods.[1]

and over the course of evolution, our bodies have adapted to be able to metabolize them efficiently.[2] Whole grains provide fiber, protein, essential fatty acids, vitamins, minerals, and numerous phytochemicals, as well as carbohydrates, in the perfect package to give us the energy we need. They have been linked to lower risk of heart disease, diabetes, obesity, certain cancers, and mortality from all causes.[3] Eating whole grains also improves bowel health, helping to maintain regular bowel movements and promote growth of healthy gut bacteria.

Contrary to popular opinion, carbs in the form of whole grains can actually help you *lose* weight. Whole grains and starchy vegetables leave you feeling full and satisfied, and therefore combat snacking and overeating, preventing you from becoming or remaining overweight.

There are so many ways to add whole grains and starchy vegetables to your daily menu. Yams and potatoes can enrich soups and stews, or be baked in the oven and served with delicious toppings. You may be accustomed to loading a baked potato with butter and cheese, but you'll be surprised at how delicious it tastes when it soaks up flavorful mushroom gravy or Smoky Bean and Root Veg Chili (see recipe, page 276). You can also make baked No-Oil Fries (see technique, page 294) and dip them in sugar-free ketchup or Simple No-Oil Hummus (see recipe, page 281). Likewise, a grilled or steamed cob of corn doesn't need to be slathered in butter to taste good. Try complementing its natural sweetness with something spicy, like chili sauce, or Cashew Sour Cream (see recipe, page 284). Squashes can be stuffed with rice and vegetables and baked for a filling one-dish meal. Grains are versatile and can be creatively used any time of day, whether it's steel-cut oatmeal for breakfast (see technique, page 265), fluffy quinoa-and-vegetable salad for lunch, or brown rice and vegetable curry for dinner. Whole grain pastas can also be a healthy choice, with delicious vegetable-based sauces.

As you find your stride as a Whole Foodie, you may want to experiment with some less familiar whole grains and starchy vegetables. Cooked buckwheat or amaranth can make a warming, nutty breakfast cereal. Ancient wheat varieties like farro, spelt, and kamut add pleasing chewy texture to salads and steamed vegetable dishes, and they are delicious cooked in soups and stews. Purple potatoes are not only beautiful but also healthful—try them with fresh herbs and a creamy plant-based dressing for a colorful twist on potato salad at your next garden party.

Cooked grains keep well in the fridge, so a practical strategy can be to batch cook—make a big pot of one of your favorites on a Sunday evening, then have it on hand all week to reheat as a bed for steamed veggies or stir-fries, to add to salads, or to warm up with fruit for a sweet morning treat. When you bake yams or potatoes, make extra—leftovers will be perfect for a breakfast hash the next morning. Frozen grains and grain medleys are quick and easy options.

2. Beans and Other Legumes

Wholesome, comforting, satisfying, and bursting with health benefits, beans and other legumes are a Whole Foodie's dream. As you shift to a whole foods, plant-based diet, you are likely to eat many more of these nourishing foods and enjoy the many benefits, hopefully daily. If you're concerned that it might get monotonous, don't be—this group of foods comprises more than thirteen hundred varieties of beans, peas, and lentils.

The legume family includes all the varieties of dried or cooked beans you can find at grocery stores: black, pinto, navy, cannellini, kidney, garbanzo (also known as chickpeas), black-eyed peas, and so on. There are also many more varieties of delicious heirloom beans that you can usually find at Whole Foods Market and other natural foods stores. Legumes also include soybeans and the foods made from them (see box, page 184). Peas and lentils in all their many colors are also legumes. Some varieties, like fava beans, lima beans, English peas, and soybeans (edamame), are eaten fresh. Green beans and snow peas fall into this category, but in these cases, because you eat the whole pod, they are better treated as a vegetable, and we include them in the "Nonstarchy Vegetables" category on page 191. Others are harvested once they have dried in their pods, and often these "mature" legumes are the most nutrient rich and delicious. Peanuts are classified as a legume, but nutritionally they behave more like a nut, so we group them with nuts and seeds and recommend consuming them in limited quantities.

Legumes are generally low-fat, high-protein, starchy foods packed with vitamins, minerals, antioxidant compounds, and dietary fiber. As you shift to a 90+% plant-based diet, you will find that these highly satiating foods are a great replacement for some of the meat you are accustomed to eating, offering many of the same beneficial nutrients without the cholesterol and saturated fat, and with the added fiber and other micronutrients found only in plant foods. Almost all varieties of legumes provide iron, zinc, B vitamins, magnesium, and potassium, among many other nutrients. Most legumes also contain significant amounts of fiber and resistant starch, which helps to regulate bowels, remove toxins, and keep blood sugar levels in check. Beans lower blood pressure[4] and reduce cholesterol.[5]

All of these factors may help to account for the fact that a taste for legumes is a common denominator among all the world's longest-lived

Is Soy Safe?

When people make the switch from a meat-heavy diet to a plant-based one, a legume that tends to take center stage on the dinner table is soy. This versatile, protein-rich food has become a favorite among vegetarians and vegans, but it has also been the subject of scares and health concerns.

The most widely held fear is that the isolates and phytoestrogens in soy may contribute to the growth of breast cancer. However, science has shown exactly the opposite: the phytoestrogens in soy appear to improve breast cancer survival rates and reduce one's risk of developing it.[8] It is important to note that these are studies where soy foods (as opposed to powders or supplements) are eaten as part of the diet. Furthermore, soy consumption may reduce the risk of prostate cancer.[9] Reviewing the science available, Dr. Neal Barnard concludes: "Evidence to date is reassuring...If you choose to include soy products in your routine, you'll have science on your side."[10]

Another common fear around soy is spurred by the fact that much of the soy grown in America today is genetically modified. While there is little conclusive evidence of harmful effects from eating GMO soybeans, the best way to minimize any possible risks is to choose organic soy products (or those marked "Non-GMO Project Verified"), which are readily available.

Our advice is to stick to traditional whole or minimally processed forms of soy. The most whole form of soy is the bean itself, which is known as edamame when eaten fresh. You may have had them as an appetizer at a Japanese restaurant. You can steam them at cultures. Remember, every single one of the Blue Zones is characterized by the presence of beans on the plate—an average of one cup per day is associated with four extra years of life expectancy. Whether it's the black-eyed peas that are a favorite in Ikaria, Greece; the soybeans eaten in Okinawa, Japan; the black beans that are a dietary staple in Nicoya, Costa Rica; the fava beans and chickpeas popular on the Italian island of Sardinia; or the

home or buy them ready shelled. They are satisfying as snacks or added to salads, stir-fries, and more. Tempeh is another whole soy food, made with fermented whole soy beans, as is miso. Try marinating tempeh and baking it in thin slices for a sandwich filling. Miso comes in several varieties, with white versions milder and red more intense. You can make miso soup (add miso at the end of cooking to avoid killing all the probiotics) or mix it with a little hot water to form a paste, which can be used in sauces and dressings.

Soy milk, tofu, and tamari are minimally processed foods, lacking much of the original fiber and nutrients in whole beans. However, they are still healthy choices that can have a place in a whole foods, plant-based diet. Choose unsweetened varieties of soy milk, and use low-sodium, MSG-free tamari or shoyu varieties of soy sauce sparingly.

If you eat soy products, treat them as a flavorful condiment— adding baked tempeh "croutons" to salad, tofu to vegetable stir-fry, or miso sauce to roasted veggies—a similar approach to that of traditional Asian diets.

Highly processed soy products, including fake meats, soy cheeses, and soy isolate protein powders, are best avoided. If you are transitioning from a meat-heavy diet to a plant-based one, they might be useful as a temporary replacement for familiar foods, but once you become comfortable building meals around whole grains, starchy vegetables, and legumes, you'll soon find you can dispense with these synthetic foods in favor of whole plant alternatives.

variety of beans on the Loma Linda, California, Adventists' plates, Buettner calls beans a "cornerstone of every longevity diet."[6] Scientists agree, having identified legume consumption as "the most important dietary predictor of survival in older people of different ethnicities."[7]

The possibilities for eating legumes are endless, and you can draw inspiration from around the globe. On a winter evening, you might enjoy Hearty Split Pea and Vegetable Soup (see recipe, page 270), or an Indian-style dal fragrant with spices, served with steaming brown basmati rice. On a hot summer day, add cold cooked beans or sprouted lentils to a salad or warm up cooked lentils with a splash of balsamic vinegar to make an earthy, protein-rich dressing. Fresh green fava beans or English peas make delicious spreads—try mashing them with fresh mint and serving on whole grain toast as an appetizer at your next dinner party. Black or pinto beans cooked (see technique, page 288) with traditional Mexican spices (see Mexican Spice Blend recipe, page 272) are a wonderful filling for tacos and burritos or a warming accompaniment to rice and vegetables. You may even enjoy the leftovers for breakfast the next day. Hummus or white bean spread is a quick and satisfying snack when paired with crunchy vegetables (see Simple No-Oil Hummus, page 281). Cooked garbanzo beans can be sprayed with liquid amino acids or soy sauce and baked for a crunchy treat.

While you may start out with the most familiar varieties, we encourage you to explore the wide range of legumes available. Don't just stick with black beans or brown lentils; try some beautiful red lentils, yellow split peas, or red kidney beans. If you're not used to eating beans or lentils, build up slowly until your body gets used to digesting them. Soaking dried beans in fresh water overnight, then tossing the water and rinsing the beans before cooking, also helps to reduce bloating and gassiness. (See page 288 for how to cook beans and lentils.) Buying beans ready cooked, although more expensive than dried beans, is a convenient option, but it's advisable to choose varieties with low sodium or no added salt, then add salt to taste when cooking if needed. Look for BPA-free cans or cartons whenever possible. However you choose to prepare them, eating legumes daily seems to be a prescription for a long and healthy life.

3. Berries

Plump blackberries. Zesty raspberries. Succulent strawberries. Juicy blueberries. Berries are some of nature's sweetest and most delicious offerings—and they're exceptionally good for you as well. We use the term *berry* in its colloquial rather than its scientific form, including all of those listed above, as well as cherries, grapes, cranberries, currants, and so on. We recommend that you eat berries regularly—perhaps every day if you enjoy them. If you have a sweet tooth, they can be a replacement for processed, sugary sweets.

A growing body of scientific evidence supports the health benefits of berries. Berries have been shown to potentially protect against cancer, and they contain high levels of ellagic acid, a compound that has been shown to inhibit the formation of tumors.[11] They also appear to protect against cognitive decline.[12] Studies have found that consuming berries daily raises "good" HDL cholesterol and lowers blood pressure, both factors associated with a lower risk of cardiovascular disease.[13] These benefits may be due to the high antioxidant content of these small but powerful fruits (see box, page 181), as berries contain more antioxidants per serving than any other food except spices.[14]

Some people worry that berries (and fruits in general) are a sugary food that should be avoided, causing diabetes and weight gain. As we discussed on page 118, these fears are misguided. Yes, berries and other fruits contain high levels of fructose, but when it comes in the form of a whole fruit, with plentiful fiber and water, fructose has a different effect on the body than it does in its isolated highly processed forms, such as high-fructose corn syrup. And if you're worried about diabetes, consider this: greater consumption of whole fruits is associated with a *lower* likelihood of developing type 2 diabetes.[15]

So go ahead and add some fresh berries to your breakfast bowl, together with a cereal like oatmeal. Or make Whole Wheat Blueberry Pancakes (see recipe, page 269). If you drink smoothies, a small handful of berries adds a boost of sweetness, a good companion for lots of greens. Berries also make a wonderful enhancement to a salad. Throw them in whole or blend a handful

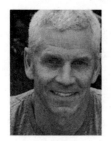

WHOLE FOODIE HERO
Rip Esselstyn

"Do you want to eat strong food or do you want to eat weak food? You've been bamboozled into thinking that steak and eggs and chicken and salmon are strong foods, when in fact they are weak foods that are insidiously destroying your health. The strong foods are the plants: they have everything you need to be the healthiest person possible."

Contributions: As a former firefighter, Rip has been the perfect messenger for the "plant-strong" movement, combating the "real men eat meat" stereotype. His profession provided the name for his Engine 2 diet and food brand—always a great choice for Whole Foodies.

Fun facts: Rip is the son of another Whole Foodie Hero, Dr. Caldwell Esselstyn.

Read this: *The Engine 2 Seven-Day Rescue Diet: Eat Plants, Lose Weight, Save Your Health*

Learn more: engine2.com

of raspberries with some white balsamic vinegar for a delicious, oil-free raspberry vinaigrette. If you crave a little after-dinner sweet, reach for a bowl of fresh strawberries or frozen cherries or grapes rather than a cookie. You can blend frozen berries with cashews and banana to make a dairy-free alternative to ice cream (see Raspberry Nice Cream, page 306).

Choose organic berries when possible because conventional varieties often receive an unhealthy dose of pesticides. Frozen berries are a good choice, retaining all the health benefits of the fresh fruit. Be careful with dried berries, such as raisins, dried currants, goji berries, or dried cranberries—although still a healthy choice, the loss of water concentrates them, making them more calorie-dense. Eat them in limited quantities, especially if weight loss is a goal.

4. Other Fruits

Besides berries, the fruit family offers a wealth of other options for you to choose from. Crunchy apples, creamy bananas, juicy peaches, exotic mangoes and papayas, zesty citrus, thirst-quenching melons—the list goes on and on. The only exceptions to our wholehearted encouragement to eat fruit are avocados and olives—both technically fruits but also high in fat, so best consumed in limited quantities when trying to lose weight. Fruits are high in fiber and contain hundreds of beneficial nutrients that support your body's functioning. They are truly one of the healthiest foods you can eat.

Humans are drawn to sweet foods for a reason—for millennia fresh fruit was the only source of natural sweetness (besides wild honey), and it came with many health benefits. Unfortunately, today that natural affinity for sweets can draw us down the wrong aisles in the supermarket. So next time you feel a craving for something sweet, remember what your ancestors would have done—choose a delicious fresh fruit. Eating fruit is a more healthful way to satisfy a sweet tooth without the weight gain that results from eating processed, refined sugars.

Enjoy fruit as often as you like—there are so many options to choose from. You can have fruit salad for breakfast, snack on an apple, add a peach to a green smoothie, make a mango salsa for tacos, toss orange slices in a salad, bake apples or apricots for a delicious dessert, grill nectarines, and even blend a frozen banana with soy milk for a whole foods, plant-based alternative to ice cream. Frozen banana slices with nut butter are a delicious dessert too.

Choose organic where possible, especially for those fruits where you eat the skin. Remember, whole fruit is always a better choice than fruit juice, which has lost its essential fiber and many other nutrients along with it, and will deliver a highly concentrated dose of sugar to your bloodstream.

5. Cruciferous Vegetables

The cruciferous family of vegetables, also known as brassica vegetables, includes broccoli, radishes, cabbage, collard greens, Brussels sprouts, cauliflower, artichokes, arugula, and kale. Not only are these diverse foods all related, they also share extraordinary health benefits, particularly for preventing cancer. Dr. Joel Fuhrman points out that cruciferous vegetables are the most micronutrient dense of all vegetables,[16] and calls them "the most powerful anticancer foods in existence." This latter distinction may be due to a potent cancer fighter that is unique and particularly important to this group of foods, a family of substances known as glucosinolates. Glucosinolates are responsible for the pungent aroma and bitter flavor of many cruciferous vegetables. When these glucosinolates are broken down (either during food preparation or through chewing and digestion), they form compounds called isothiocyanates and indoles that have been shown in numerous studies to inhibit the development of cancer.[17]

Despite their outsize health benefits, cruciferous vegetables often play only a minor role in American diets. Many associate broccoli and cabbage with their least favorite childhood meals, and while kale has gotten press the last few years as a "superfood," many people don't know how to prepare it in ways that are tasty or without lots of oil.

It turns out moms all over America are right when they tell kids, "Eat your broccoli"! The good news is there are many creative ways to eat broccoli and other cruciferous vegetables that your mom may not have known about. Raw or lightly steamed broccoli or cauliflower florets provide satisfying crunch to salads and on their own when dipped in hummus. Kale can be blended raw into smoothies, "massaged" into a salad (see Kale Waldorf Salad, page 280), or lightly steamed with garlic and lemon juice. Zesty radishes, thinly sliced, add bite to salads, while the peppery flavor of arugula makes a nice change from lettuce. Toss a few handfuls into warm pasta with veggies. Bok choy is a lovely addition to stir-fries, with its combination of crunchy stalks and tender leaves. Add it right at the end of cooking, as it needs only a couple of minutes.

6. Leafy Greens

Remember Dr. Joel Fuhrman's formula for health? Eat as many micronutrients as possible while not consuming excess calories. By this measure of "nutrient density," the undisputed winners are leafy greens.

Some of the top-scoring greens also fall into the cruciferous category—kale, collards, arugula, and bok choy. Other particularly potent greens include watercress, Swiss chard, spinach, romaine, and other salad greens.

Researchers at Harvard University found greens to be the food most highly associated with protection from major chronic disease and cardiovascular disease.[18] They have also been associated with reduced risk of diabetes.[19] Greens are packed with fiber, protein, and antioxidants, as well as a long list of vitamins, minerals, and disease-fighting phytochemicals.

You can eat greens raw as a salad, add handfuls to a smoothie, steam them lightly and serve them with lemon juice, toss them into soup or stew at the end of cooking to lightly wilt, blend them into flavorful pesto-style sauces (see recipe, page 299), add steamed greens to mashed potatoes, or water-sauté them with garlic. Spinach is a nutrient-rich addition to homemade hummus or other bean spreads. Greens are so extraordinarily healthful that we add them whenever possible to the dishes we cook. Try to eat greens every day.

7. Nonstarchy Vegetables

Only about one in ten Americans eats enough fruits and vegetables, according to a recent government report.[20] One estimate, from the Union of Concerned Scientists, says that if Americans ate just one more serving of fruits and vegetables daily it would save more than thirty thousand lives annually, and billions of dollars in medical costs.[21] No matter how many points nutritionists and dietary experts seem to argue about, this is the one that they universally agree upon: *eat more vegetables!* We've already discussed several distinct categories of vegetables, so this category simply encompasses the wonderful variety not accounted for in previous mention: zucchini, carrots, peppers, mushrooms, green beans, onions, eggplants, celery, asparagus, and many, many more. Each of these vegetables has its own store of health benefits, too many to list here, but here are a few tips for ensuring you get as many of them as possible:

Eat the rainbow. Colorful vegetables tend to contain the most antioxidants, and where antioxidants go, health tends to follow. Brighten your plate and eat as many different colors as possible.

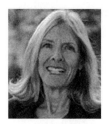

WHOLE FOODIE HERO
Mary McDougall

"Although the McDougall Diet includes thousands of recipes, we eat very simply and suggest you do the same. A typical breakfast is oatmeal with blueberries. For dinner we have a flavorful bean stew cooked in my crockpot over boiled potatoes, just plain baked sweet potatoes, or mashed potatoes made in my Instant Pot with my creamy golden gravy. You can tell we love potatoes!"

Contribution: Nutritional science is important, but the rubber meets the road in the kitchen. Preparing food, stocking a pantry, creating delicious recipes, and building an entire Whole Foodie lifestyle is just as essential. Mary McDougall—best-selling author, teacher, coach, and partner at Dr. McDougall's Health and Medical Center—has been a leader and pioneer in this regard, creating over three thousand recipes and influencing people around the world with optimum lifestyle practices.

Read this: *The New McDougall Cookbook*

Learn more: drmcdougall.com

Don't neglect the less colorful ones. For example, mushrooms, garlic, and onions are packed with beneficial nutrients, and all are potent immune-supporting and anticancer foods. Dr. Fuhrman advises cooking mushrooms to avoid potential toxins in raw form.[22]

Add a vegetable! Whenever you cook one of the other categories of food, ask yourself if you could add some more veggies. Lentil soup? Add carrots, tomatoes, zucchini, or a few handfuls of greens. Tomato sauce? Add mushrooms or bell peppers. Brown rice? Make it a rice pilaf with a variety of chopped steamed veggies and fresh herbs.

You can prepare side dishes with individual vegetables, but some recipes allow you to combine multiple vegetables. Try an oil-free vegetable stir-fry with colorful peppers, crunchy bok choy, and earthy shiitake mushrooms. Or make a

MY WHOLE FOODIE STORY

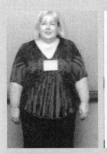
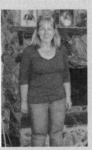

Debbie Schafer, 52, Dallas, Texas
Switching to a whole foods, plant-based diet changed my life forever. I used to wear a size twenty-four, and took blood pressure meds, heartburn meds, and allergy meds. In October 2012, I was given the opportunity to attend a weeklong Immersion program with Dr. Joel Fuhrman. In the year that followed, I lost more than 125 pounds, got off all my meds, and now wear a size ten. My transformation story was featured on the cover of *Woman's World* magazine. At age fifty-two, I feel better than I did in my twenties, and I can almost keep up with my six-year-old granddaughter!

vibrant pasta salad with steamed broccoli, peppers, green beans, and asparagus. Salads can quickly turn into delicious and nutritious whole meals with the addition of raw or steamed veggies and a handful of whole grains and beans. Soups combine a variety of vegetables, along with beans as well. A mixed platter of raw sliced vegetables with hummus or a dip is a great party food that can help you resist reaching for the corn chips. The bottom line when it comes to vegetables: however you enjoy them, eat them. Then eat some more!

8. Nuts and Seeds

Nuts and seeds round out our list of essential whole foods to enjoy daily. We feel these are an important category of foods for many reasons. The simplest, of course, is that nuts and seeds are packed with health-promoting nutrients and are consistently associated with good health outcomes. They are a rich source of many nutrients—understandable, given that they contain the energy to create an entire plant or tree.

Indeed, the consumption of nuts and seeds has been associated with reduced risk of heart disease and diabetes, as well as an increased life span.[23] In the Blue Zones, centenarians regularly consume about a handful (around two ounces) of varying types of nuts per day. The Adventist Health Studies also point to impressive benefits, with nut-eaters living longer by a couple of years than those who don't eat nuts.[24] While some people raise concerns about the relatively high calorie density of nuts, they are also extremely filling and generally *not* associated with an increase in weight or BMI.[25] Having said that, if you are trying to lose weight, limit nut and seed intake to less than a handful a day.

This category of food also contains some of the most concentrated plant sources of essential omega-3 fatty acids. The body cannot make these important nutrients, so we have to get them from food or supplements (see page 175). Although many whole plant foods contain small amounts of omega-3 fatty acids, some nuts and seeds, such as flaxseeds, chia seeds, hemp seeds, and walnuts, contain particularly high amounts.

Nuts and seeds can easily be mixed into your favorite foods. Sprinkle a few chopped almonds on morning oatmeal or add them to salads. Nuts can be blended with fresh herbs to make a salad dressing or creamy pesto (see Oil-Free Herb Pesto, page 299). Cashews, soaked overnight, can be blended into creamy sauces (see Cashew Sour Cream, page 284), dressings, or desserts. Ground flaxseeds or hemp seed are easily added to smoothies, sprinkled over breakfast cereal or oatmeal, or baked in muffins. Flaxseeds and chia seeds have a "binding" quality, and are ideal for thickening sauces or replacing eggs in baking. Similarly, chia seeds bind together and take on liquid. Soak them in a little soy or almond milk to make a creamy pudding, which you can sweeten by adding mashed bananas, berries, or other fruits.

CHAPTER 11

Healthier *and* Happier

The Psychology and Physiology of Food and Pleasure

"We take it for granted that our feelings are what they are and cannot be
altered…that we do not have a choice, when in fact we do."

—*Tal Ben-Shahar, Choose the Life You Want*

Good food is one of life's greatest pleasures. The anticipation of a favorite
meal; the first taste of a tender, perfectly prepared dish; the subtle flavors of
herbs; the warmth and camaraderie of breaking bread with those we love;
the feeling of fullness when all is done. The human palate is an extraordinary
gift; its thousands of taste buds deliver myriad pleasurable sensations and
inspire the human race's unrivaled culinary creativity.

Some of us love the exquisite pain of fiery spices; others relish the tangy
freshness of citrus or fermented foods; others savor rich, salty, or pungent fare;
and still others cherish the soothing touch of sweetness. As we eat the foods
we love, we enjoy not only the immediate flavors that tantalize our senses, but
also the reawakened memories of past pleasures shared with family, friends,
and community. Food preferences are a highly personal matter, interwoven
with a sense of identity and culture. Many of us, when we consider changing
our diet, fear that we will lose all of this. Many people will do anything—
exercise intensely, take pills, even go under the surgeon's knife—before they
will consider changing what's on their plates. We guard our relationship with
food like a jealous lover. Science may convince us that change is a good idea,

continued on page 198

MY WHOLE FOODIE STORY

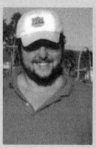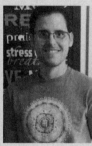

**Adam Sud, 34,
Santa Monica, California**
Four years ago I checked into rehab.
I was addicted to Adderal, weighed
more than three hundred pounds,
typically ate six cheeseburgers
a day, and suffered from severe
depression. My relationships with
my family and friends had become strained, and I was barely working
and fast running out of money. I knew I needed help, and fast.

A year earlier I had attended Rip Esselstyn's Engine 2 Immersion,
but in the grip of my addiction, I wasn't ready to make the change.

On my first day of rehab, I found out I had type 2 diabetes. I was
prescribed no fewer than seven medications—including diabetes
medications, blood pressure medications, sleeping pills, ADHD drugs,
bipolar medications, and more. I looked at my weight and my blood
sugar numbers and I knew I'd done that to myself. So I decided, *If I
was the cause of my problems, then I'm going to be the solution.*

When I got out of rehab, I went into sober living and immediately
adopted a plant-based lifestyle. In three months I reversed my
diabetes. Plant-based nutrition became the backbone of my entire
recovery. Within one year I was off all seven medications. Today I am
over four years sober and weigh 160 pounds. I lost 160 pounds. My
waist size has gone from forty-seven inches to thirty-one.

I won't say the transition was easy. I'm a seventh-generation Texan
who grew up eating burgers and barbeque. Going from that to
eating kale is tough, so I told myself over and over that I had to get
comfortable with being uncomfortable. I knew that for a while I
would have to wake up each day and do things I didn't want to do.
But the alternative was that I was probably going to die.

For me, one of the keys was simplicity. I basically ate the same
meals every day for ten months. Oatmeal for breakfast. Beans,
greens, corn, veggies, and marinara sauce for lunch. Lots of fruit
throughout the day. People often get intimidated by the idea that

they have to learn so many different new meals. I tell them, just find one or two you like and start with those.

These days I make epic salads with baked sweet potatoes, and I can't wait to eat them. I eat more than I ever ate before. When you make a meal that's aimed at creating health and wellness, that's an act of self-care. It's about creating a better version of yourself today than you were yesterday. That is the essence of recovery. It builds self-worth, and when you have self-worth you feel like you're worth saving every day. Recovery is not just abstinence—it's about finding new things to validate your life. These days I'm addicted to my plant-based lifestyle!

I have a twin brother, who at the end of last year was right about where I had been, minus the drug addiction. He weighed more than 250 pounds, had type 2 diabetes, high blood pressure, and high cholesterol, and was depressed. I said to him, "I'm not judging you, but are you happy the way you are?" He said no. I asked him if he could afford to take six months off and move in with me and live my lifestyle, and he agreed.

He started eating the same diet I ate, and taking walks in the mornings. In just one week, his blood sugar dropped lower than he'd ever been able to get it with medications. In three weeks his blood pressure dropped to normal. And in two and a half months he lost more than forty pounds. He's gotten off his diabetes meds and blood pressure meds, and is slowly weaning himself off his antidepressants. I can see the light starting to come on in his eyes.

As for me, I've become a certified holistic lifestyle coach and developed a program to use nutrition as a tool for addiction recovery and relapse prevention. I enjoy telling people about all the weight I've lost and the meds I threw out, but even more than that, I love telling them what I have gained: a real relationship with my family; a purpose in life; a sense of self-worth and self-confidence; an ability to help others. Everything about the way that I think, feel, and move through the world has changed as a result of this. I have never been happier or healthier. Plant-based eating didn't just save my life; it gave me an entirely new life.

continued from page 195

but science alone won't persuade us to actually transform what we're eating, because when it comes to food, we tend to be more emotional than rational. Food is a significant source of happiness in life, and no diet that deprives us of that pleasure for too long is ultimately sustainable.

It goes without saying, then, that to successfully shift eating habits we need to ensure that the new foods are delicious. However, it's not quite that simple. If you have ever tried to significantly change your diet, you know that it is as much a psychological challenge as it is a physical one. Therefore, it's helpful to understand a few basic principles about human psychology and physiology as they relate to food, pleasure, and habit change.

First, it's important to recognize that the relationship between food and pleasure has been complicated by the environment in which most of us live, with its overabundance of highly processed foods and the majority of people around you condoning their consumption as normal. Second, it helps to remember that any kind of change is a process that takes time. Understanding the dynamics of this process, and the stages through which you will pass, can give you the patience and motivation to stick with it for long enough to reap the rewards. We've each made this transition ourselves, and have supported thousands of others—friends, loved ones, team members, and patients. In the pages that follow, we'll share some of the insights that we've found most helpful on the journey.

Escaping the Pleasure Trap

"In human and in animal life, the primary goals are the pursuit of pleasure, the avoidance of pain, and the conservation of energy," declare psychologist Doug Lisle, PhD, and Alan Goldhamer, DC, in their book *The Pleasure Trap: Mastering the Hidden Force That Undermines Health and Happiness.* "Pleasure was designed as the unmistakable signal of success for reaching survival and/ or reproductive goals."[1] Lisle and Goldhamer have been extremely influential in elucidating the human relationship with food.

Pleasure—particularly in the form of a brain chemical called dopamine—played an important evolutionary role in ensuring that humans ate enough to survive and had sex in order to reproduce. But in our modern environment, where we can get an easy pleasure "hit" from drugs or from druglike highly processed foods, it's become a less trustworthy signal. "The natural internal compass of life's decision-making can be deceived," they write. Because "feeling good is a hallmark of biological success,"[2] intense and easy experiences of pleasure trick us into believing that something valuable is happening, when in fact, we may be doing great damage to our bodies and minds. Lisle and Goldhamer call this "the pleasure trap."

One core insight of *The Pleasure Trap* is that highly processed foods work in similar ways to addictive drugs. This is not just an analogy—studies have shown that the body's response to drugs like heroin, cocaine, nicotine, or alcohol is identical to its response to food.[3] You may think you crave chocolate for its taste, but researchers have demonstrated that in fact, when people are given an opiate blocker that impedes the druglike effect, they are much less likely to devour a bar of chocolate. What they were really craving was the stimulation of emotional and physical pleasure.[4] And it's not just chocolate. Studies have come to similar conclusions about dairy products, finding that they contain a protein called casein that breaks down in the body into casomorphin, a mild opiate.[5] Knowing this makes it easy to understand why we love dairy, and cheese in particular—it has more concentrated amounts of casein than milk, ice cream, or butter.

The problem with drugs, as Lisle and Goldhamer explain, is that they quickly dull sensitivity to subtle pleasures. As long as we don't take drugs, our bodies have a normal baseline of arousal. Once people begin to take drugs regularly, they find themselves in a heightened state of arousal that over time becomes the norm. Then when we stop taking drugs, we go through withdrawal and have terrible lows as our body readjusts to a normal baseline state of arousal. In the same way, "People consuming a diet of whole natural foods will experience a normal range of pleasure chemistry activation," Lisle and Goldhamer write. However, if highly processed druglike foods are consumed regularly, a process known as neuroadaptation will take place. Initially we'll experience those foods as being more pleasurable than the whole food alternatives. We'll begin to enjoy the bigger dopamine surges and start acclimating to that greater "high." Over time "the taste nerves adapt to this higher level of stimulation, a process that is barely noticeable. Later, we may believe that we are enjoying the rich diet more than a simpler, health-promoting diet, but this is an illusion."[6] In other words, *whatever diet we consume regularly will begin to taste better to us and provide a similar level of arousal.*

Once those higher levels of stimulation begin to feel normal (through the process of neuroadaptation), when we go back to eating healthier foods with a lower dopamine surge, we may feel exceptionally "low." Like drug addicts who can no longer experience the simple joys of life without the artificial stimulation of a cocktail of chemicals, food addicts cannot appreciate the delights of nature's bounty until the food has been unnaturally concentrated or adulterated with fat, salt, and sugar. They are caught in the "pleasure trap," and convinced that they will never enjoy eating again if they give up highly processed favorites and replace them with whole foods.

So can we escape the pleasure trap? Yes, we can. Our bodies can acclimate back to our normal baseline—it just takes a little time and the right food choices. To understand how this works, think about what happens when you spend time outside on a really hot day. At first it may be unbearable, but eventually your body may adjust and it will feel normal. When you step into the shade it feels cooler, and when you step into an air-conditioned room, it may even feel cold. After some time in the air-conditioned room, you begin to acclimate, and now that feels normal. If you step outside, it will feel too hot again. The body acclimates to food in a similar way, although it takes longer. The key is to give our palates time to readapt. Lisle and Goldhamer recommend allowing thirty to ninety days for that neuroadaptation to take place and for the palate to become resensitized to the more subtle pleasures of eating whole, natural foods.

During this period it's critical to know what's going on in your body and to expect that your eating experience may be challenging and feel less pleasurable. When we decrease the calorie density of our foods by choosing whole foods, and mostly plants, we will initially decrease the stimulation derived from foods. This is why it's so important to eat enough so we don't add to the problem by not getting enough calories.

Even if we are careful to eat enough calories, some people may still feel withdrawal from addictive, concentrated, processed foods and the stimulation they provide. The experience of stimulation is dropping back to a more normal level, but that drop may feel like a physical crash similar to that of cutting down or eliminating caffeine or another addictive drug. It can make us feel tired, anxious, and miserable. And most of all, it makes us desperate for another dopamine hit—one that will get us back to our heightened state of arousal.

Understanding this process that is taking place inside your body can be reassuring when you're in the midst of it. You can remind yourself that after an initial resensitization period, your pleasure receptors and dopamine levels will reach their baseline once again, ultimately giving you the exact level of pleasure you had when eating highly processed foods. Plus, once your palate has normalized, you will be able to taste subtle flavors of foods that you couldn't taste before because your taste buds were overwhelmed with the greater stimulation of processed foods. You'll enjoy another highly pleasurable experience: the feeling of greater energy and vitality that health-promoting foods bestow. Reminding yourself of these benefits to come can ease the discomfort of withdrawal to some degree. But that doesn't mean it will be easy, especially at first.

The good news is that, unlike traditional dieting, which relies on calorie restriction, shifting to a whole foods, plant-based diet gets easier, not harder, as you go on. As with learning a new language, the more you immerse yourself in the life and culture, the faster you become fluent. You'll become a skillful eater—developing better and more efficient systems to keep yourself nourished and satisfied. And your taste buds will develop, so you start to love the foods that love you right back—whole plant foods.

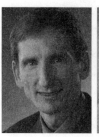 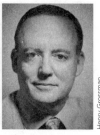

WHOLE FOODIE HEROES
Doug Lisle, PhD, and Alan Goldhamer, DC

Henry Grossman

"The march of history is that of the human race obeying the mantra of the motivational triad—attempting to attain more pleasure, for less pain, with ever-greater efficiency."

Contributions: Lisle and Goldhamer are long-term partners in working at the intersection of food and psychology. Goldhamer founded the TrueNorth Health Center in Northern California, where Lisle joined him in 1997. Their book *The Pleasure Trap* is one of the most insightful works on human motivation and diet.

Fun facts: Lisle and Goldhamer were childhood best friends, and Lisle's initial interest in diet and health, as well as his adoption of a plant-based diet, was inspired by Goldhamer.

Read this: *The Pleasure Trap: Mastering the Hidden Force that Undermines Health and Happiness*

Learn more: healthpromoting.com

Dealing with Deprivation

The word *diet* does not hold positive associations for most of us. In the minds of many, it is inseparable from another dreaded *D*-word, *deprivation*. Most diets rely on portion control, achieved through willpower. Not only is this a very unpleasant way to live, it's also quite ineffective. The feeling of deprivation that comes with portion control often makes people more likely to binge on calorie-dense foods.

Deprivation is not just an emotional experience you can ignore—it's also physiological. Your body has a system for letting you know when you've eaten enough, which includes the release of a hormone called leptin. When you don't eat enough, because you're desperately practicing portion control, your

Eat Your Way to Happiness

It may come as no surprise that certain foods can increase feelings of happiness. But what may surprise you is that we're not talking about chocolate or bacon. In fact, the foods most positively associated with psychological well-being are...fruits and vegetables! Studies from around the world show that people who have high daily fruit and vegetable intakes are more likely to be classified as very happy.[7] In one large study conducted in Great Britain, it was found that the more fruits and vegetables people ate, the higher they rated their life satisfaction and happiness. Researchers controlled for many factors that could have explained away the result, and still came up with a significant correlation.[8] Another study found that those eating more fruits and vegetables reported greater feelings of engagement, meaning, purpose, curiosity, and creativity.[9]

Of course, as Dr. Michael Greger points out in a video on the topic,[10] causation could go either way. "Which came first, the mood or the food?" he asks. However, one study he cites did indeed show a correlation between eating fruits and vegetables one day, and feeling better the next.[11] So if you need more reasons to eat more fruits and veggies than we've given you in this book so far, do it to keep the blues away!

body won't release that hormone, and you'll continue to feel hungry. In fact, you'll feel even stronger cravings for calorie-dense food because your body feels it needs to make up for a deficit. When you deprive yourself of adequate nourishment, you're working against your body's natural instincts. And eventually your starving body will overcome your best intentions to "be good" through willpower, resulting in the binge cycle that dieters know all too well.

Think of this transition to becoming a Whole Foodie as a lifestyle change rather than a diet. Remember, you should feel full and satisfied after you eat, and because you're eating foods that are less calorie dense, you'll be able to eat *more*, not less. Don't make the mistake of going hungry and increasing the likelihood you'll experience feelings of deprivation.

If you eat whole foods, plant-based meals that include plenty of satiating foods like whole grains, starchy vegetables, and beans and other legumes, you should be able to mitigate the unpleasant experience of "dieting" to a significant degree. When your diet can include healthy versions of your favorite foods, like pancakes, baked potatoes, stir-fries, cookies, even pizza, it feels less like a diet. However, in the early stages of a transition, you may struggle with cravings. Challenge yourself to fulfill those cravings in a healthy manner (see page 211). If you ensure that you give your body adequate nourishment in the form of

If Hunger Is Not the Problem, Eating Is Not the Solution

Many motivations can lead us to stimulating foods—and many of them have little to do with hunger. These include anxiety, depression, stress, loneliness, tiredness, and boredom. These conditions sometimes cause us to eat to make ourselves feel better—to get the dopamine pleasure hit that will temporarily numb the uncomfortable or painful feelings. We reach for "comfort foods"—chocolate, cookies, pizza, doughnuts, potato chips, macaroni and cheese, and so on. And we never choose broccoli!

The problem with comfort eating, besides unhealthy foods, is that because motivations have nothing to do with true hunger, eating does little to appease them in the long term. To make things worse, it actually adds to the emotional burden by luring us back into the diet trap: we overeat, gain weight, panic, go on a diet, feel deprived and miserable, binge, then start all over again. This is why it's so important to be mindful of what's driving your cravings. If it's not hunger, food won't fill the hole. Just pausing to drink a full glass of water and assess what you really need can make a big difference in the decision you make next. And if you do decide to reach for a comfort food, which we all do once in a while, try to make it a healthier, whole food version.

If you find yourself "comfort eating" regularly, it may be an indicator that some unacknowledged emotion or unmet need is lurking below the surface. Imagine you are wearing a pair of shoes whole plant foods, you'll start to retrain your instincts. Over time you will acclimate to the new foods and soon you'll find yourself craving those!

How Your Tastes Can Evolve

If you're struggling with the experience of new foods, here's the good news: Tastes are not innate; they are acquired. You've developed them over a lifetime of eating certain types of food—particularly the salty, fatty, or

that you love, but they are tight and hurting your feet. Instead of changing your shoes, you go get a back massage, which makes you temporarily feel good, but doesn't do anything to address the underlying issue, the tight shoes. It may distract you momentarily from your discomfort, but you'll continue to feel worse over the long term.

Try to be mindful of the wider range of your emotional needs, instead of seeking the illusory quick fix of pleasure. Maybe you need more support because you feel overwhelmed. Maybe you're feeling deprived of pleasure, lonely, or overstressed. Taking the time to identify the real problem allows you to determine a behavior strategy focused on meeting your actual needs.

When emotional needs come to the surface, don't ignore them. Instead welcome them and try to find a constructive way to approach them; no matter how much willpower you have, you won't be able to resist them indefinitely. Sometimes it is necessary to experience a few diet and lifestyle indiscretions in order to get to know yourself and ensure you're taking a holistic approach to your own emotional life. There is a lot to learn when you "fall off the wagon"—both what not to do and what to do more of. Remember, the only way to truly fail is to not get up and try again.

Learning to identify your needs in this way will allow you to take a more compassionate approach to yourself, even at those moments when you are less than perfect, and create strategies that meet more of your needs without compromising your helalth.

sugary ones—and that means they can also change over time thanks to the process of neuroadaptation (see page 200).

It won't happen overnight—your new plant-based foods may initially seem bland in comparison to the highly processed foods you're accustomed to. You may even need to use a little extra seasoning or salt at first. But over a period of weeks, you will start to adjust to the subtler flavors and enjoy your new menus.

Dr. Joel Fuhrman says that you need to exercise your palate, stretch your taste buds. It may take several tries before you begin to appreciate something unusual or different from your normal fare. Taste is influenced by familiarity, so as you get to know a new food you may find your affection for it growing. Don't overwhelm yourself with new and unfamiliar foods when you're just beginning to make a change—start slowly, with the most familiar. Skillful eating is about giving health-promoting foods a chance; find out which ones you love, then focus on those, making those meals your easiest options.

CHAPTER 12

Making the Shift

Proven Strategies for Successful Transitions

"You can't go back and make a new start, but you can start right now
and make a brand-new ending."

—*James R. Sherman, Rejection*

Over the past decades, we've each seen thousands of people successfully
transition to a whole foods, plant-based diet. In this chapter we'll share
some of the most valuable strategies we've developed and discovered for
making the transition smoothly and successfully. Some of these we created
ourselves; others represent best practices we've learned from the remarkable
community of dedicated doctors, nutritionists, health coaches, and chefs
who are working to promote this important shift.

Find Your Pace

The Whole Foods Diet is not a short-term cleanse or weight-loss program—
it's a lifestyle change that we hope will last you the rest of a very long and
healthy lifetime. So it's important to take the time you need to make the
transition, sustainably, in the way that works best for you. A gradual, staged
transition will be the most effective path for some people, while going all
in, all at once might be best for others. Different personality types require
different strategies. You also need to take into account your particular health
circumstances, and the kind of diet and lifestyle you're accustomed to. Most

importantly, it's what you are truly willing to do right now, whether that is reviewing the recipe section in Part III of this book, experimenting with changing your diet one day a week, or committing to following the 28-Day Eat Real Food Plan.

If you decide to stage your transition, consider a strategy like changing one daily meal each week to a whole foods, plant-based one—starting with breakfast, then lunch, then dinner. This is the strategy Alona and Matt use in *The Forks over Knives Plan: How to Transition to the Life-Saving, Whole-Food, Plant-Based Diet*, and it's worked very well for many people. Or you might focus your first week or two on eliminating processed foods and then scale down or phase out your consumption of animal foods over several weeks.

If you decide to go all in, the 28-Day Eat Real Food Plan in chapter 14 has been designed to guide and support you through four weeks of whole foods, plant-based eating.

Either way, give yourself time to adjust and have confidence that your food preferences can change—sometimes dramatically (see chapter 11). Many people assume that they will always crave certain types of salty, fatty, sugary foods—when they think about dietary changes, they imagine a lifetime of self-deprivation, not realizing that, given time to adjust, their bodies will eventually enjoy more wholesome fare. Psychologist Daniel Gilbert has written in depth about how terrible human beings are at predicting what will make them happy in the future. We spend our lives imagining and planning for what we think our future selves will like or dislike, then when we get there, we don't feel the way we thought we would feel. Gilbert suggests that instead of putting so much faith in power of prediction, which so often turns out wrong, we should appreciate our amazing ability to adapt to the new and unexpected.

We encourage you not to spend too much time thinking about the long term at this moment. Don't try to plan the rest of your life on the Whole Foods Diet: just think about the next week or the next month. Pick a pace you're confident you can stick with—where you can make steady progress. You can always speed up if you gain momentum. Ideally, you will create new habits, one ritual at a time. The goal is for the ritual of eating whole plant foods three times per day to become as solidified in your life as the daily ritual of brushing your teeth or combing your hair.

Know Your Why

As with any significant shift, it's important to be prepared. Preparation doesn't just mean making a shopping list or buying a cookbook. As Thomas Campbell, MD, coauthor of *The China Study*, writes, "When you're thinking of radically revising something as significant as your daily eating habits, it's worth taking stock of your head and heart before jumping into the kitchen."[1] That taking stock starts with your why.

There are many reasons for embracing a lifestyle change like the Whole Foods Diet. As you prepare to make your transition, it's important to know yours. Perhaps your doctor gave you some scary numbers, and you need to make changes before it's too late. Maybe you are trying to lose weight and improve your general sense of vitality and well-being. Maybe you are thinking of it as upping the odds that you will be active and thriving well into your old age. A friend, a book, or a movie may have convinced you to give it a go. You may already be suffering from a chronic condition like heart disease or diabetes and want to reverse it and get off your medications. Or perhaps someone you love needs to make this transition and you've decided to support him or her on this journey. You could have decided for ethical reasons that you no longer want to eat animal foods.

All of these are worthy reasons to make the shift. Embrace your reason for doing so and take full responsibility for it. Even if circumstances beyond your control have brought you to this step, it's still yours to take or not. Take time to think about the outcomes you'd like to see—not just the bad things you want to avoid, like a heart attack, but the positive things you'll gain. Envision what you'll do with your longer, healthier life—the grandchildren you'll see grow up, the retirement you'll be able to enjoy, the places in the world you may travel if you're fit and vital into old age. Think of the athletic

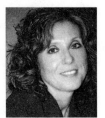

WHOLE FOODIE HERO
Pam Popper, PhD, ND

"[As Americans], we've eaten ourselves into the dubious distinction of being the fattest population in recorded history. Now we've got to figure out how we're going to teach more than three hundred million people to eat their way out of this terrible state."

Contributions: In addition to being a *New York Times* best-selling author and speaker, Popper is founder of Wellness Forum Health, a healthcare clinic, nutritional center, and educational center, all dedicated to promoting health and wellness while turning back the clock on chronic disease.

Fun facts: Popper has worked and taught with T. Colin Campbell in his nutritional courses at Cornell, and has testified in Washington as an advocate of plant-based medicine and patient rights.

Read this: *Food Over Medicine: The Conversation That Could Save Your Life*

Learn more: drpampopper.com

goals that may be in reach if you're able to reach an ideal weight. Imagine the peace of mind you'll feel when you establish a sustainable way of eating that doesn't involve constant self-deprivation or struggle. All of these benefits of change are gifts to yourself when you choose to adopt a whole foods, plant-based diet. Be accountable for your choice to do so. In a few weeks, you will thank yourself!

Eat Enough!

One of the most common reasons people struggle in the transition to a whole foods, plant-based diet is that they don't eat enough. That's right. You're much more likely to fail from eating too little than from eating too much. Many people start out by focusing on what they shouldn't eat and don't give enough attention to all the good things they *should* be eating. Because whole plant foods are less calorie dense than highly processed foods and animal foods, you may need to eat larger portions or more frequently than you are accustomed to. Try to include as many of the Essential Eight (see chapter 10) in your everyday diet as possible, and particularly focus on starchy vegetables, whole grains, and legumes.

Listen to your body, especially in the early days of your transition. If you feel hungry again only a couple hours after eating, you probably didn't have a big enough meal or include enough satiating whole grains or starchy vegetables. If you feel satisfied and content, stop eating, but if not, eat more. There is no right or wrong time to eat, only right and wrong foods. You can now trust your hunger signals without fear of overconsuming calories. You're no longer in a battle with your body or your cravings—so long as the only food on your plate is real food (particularly of the whole foods, plant-based variety).

Redirect Your Cravings

How do we deal with cravings? Too often, on traditional calorie-restriction diets, people resist and resist and resist, using willpower, until eventually they give in and binge. And then they feel bad. Over time, this cycle causes weight gain.

Ignoring cravings doesn't work very well—in fact, it tends to inflame them. As Mark Twain said, "There is a charm about the forbidden that makes it unspeakably desirable." Don't panic when cravings hit. Take a deep breath, then be mindful of your cravings in order to learn what particular flavors you need to include in your new diet. Challenge yourself to include them in a healthy way! This does *not* mean substituting broccoli for chocolate and brown rice for burgers and French fries. This *does* mean making veggie burgers with baked potato fries. Or mixing unsweetened cocoa, dates, avocados, and almond milk together to make chocolate pudding. The same goes for pizza, pasta, lasagna, cookies, cakes, and so on. A healthier version exists for almost all foods.

Longing for corn chips and guacamole? Make some easy, oil-free tortilla chips (see technique, page 273) or replace the chips with some crunchy raw vegetables. Missing your favorite ice cream? Blend up frozen fruits with cashews or unsweetened plant milk (see Raspberry Nice Cream, page 306), and add unsweetened cocoa if you crave chocolate. Wishing you could grab a soda on a hot day? Blend some frozen berries into a puree, then add sparkling water. It's perfectly natural to crave the foods you've been accustomed to eating all your life, especially at first. This is why it's important to build your transition around the foods you love—but in new, healthier versions.

Crowd Out

One of our favorite terms from the world of nutrition is "crowd out." It simply means this: fill up your plate, and your stomach, with the good stuff and there won't be much space left for anything else. Again the focus is shifted from what you *shouldn't* eat—"cutting out"—to what you *should* eat. As Kathy Freston suggests in her entertaining and highly informative *The Book of Veganish*, "think of it as swapping foods out rather than 'giving things up.' It'll be more fun that way! After all, you're eliminating certain foods from your diet in order to make room for a whole new world of delicious veggies, whole grains, and other veganish treats."[2]

A simple strategy for crowding out is to eat a big salad as your first course, or a big bowl of fruit at breakfast. Fill up on greens, veggies, or fruit before you move on to more calorie-dense foods.

Plan Ahead

Another important piece of advice is to make these healthier foods in advance. Don't wait for the craving to come on—that's not the time to start fixing things in the kitchen. Have these foods readily available whenever cravings hit. You may not know exactly what you will crave, but you can probably predict your patterns.

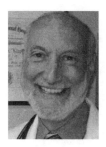

WHOLE FOODIE HERO
Michael Klaper, MD

"The vast majority of infections, inflammations, and various dysfunctions do not require high-tech interventions or expensive therapies. Successful healing requires discovering and ameliorating the true cause of these problems."

Contributions: Dr. Klaper has been a prominent advocate of plant-based nutrition for decades. Currently on the staff of TrueNorth Health Center in Santa Rosa, California, he has served in a number of executive and advisory capacities, been a consultant to NASA, and for eleven years, hosted a radio program on health and healing broadcast in Hawaii and Washington, DC.

Fun facts: A humane and deeply spiritual man, Dr. Klaper combines his medical practice with an ethical vegan lifestyle and a regular yoga and fitness regimen. He was honored with the Courage of Conscience Award from the prestigious Peace Abbey Foundation.

Learn more: DoctorKlaper.com

Doug Lisle and Alan Goldhamer explain that humans have evolved to conserve energy by taking the path of least resistance, and choosing the easiest option. Unfortunately, in contemporary America, the path of least resistance generally leads away from health and longevity. This is why it's so critical to plan and create strategies to make healthy whole food choices easy. Remember how the Blue Zones were built on "nudges and defaults"—with the healthiest options being the most convenient ones?

If you follow the 28-Day Eat Real Food Plan, we've made this part easy for you. Working with a professionally designed meal plan and recipes means you'll always know what to buy, what to cook, and what to eat—and you can be confident you are getting a rich variety of whole foods to nourish your body and meet its needs. However, we hope you'll keep going beyond

Three-Stage Eating

A really helpful way to practice the crowding-out principle is to eat your meal in three courses. Courses one and two are mandatory, course three is optional.

First course: Fruits or vegetables. This is your "weight-loss medicine and multivitamin." Whether it's a bowl of berries or other fruit before breakfast, a salad with steamed veggies before lunch, or a vegetable soup before dinner, make sure you eat a big portion.

Second course: Highly satiating whole foods like whole grains, starchy vegetables, and beans. Think of this one as your "filler" and eat a large portion.

Third course: More rich or calorie-dense foods (nuts, seeds, avocados, olives, dried fruit), minimally processed foods (whole grain pastas or bread, nut milks, tofu), animal foods (if you are including these in your diet), and so on. This course is optional— if you're already full and don't need this, that's great! If you do eat it, keep the portion smaller. And before having seconds of course three, be sure to have seconds of one and two.

Once eating this way becomes second nature, you can put all the food on one plate, but the three-course system is a great way to train yourself to be mindful and get your priorities right.

the twenty-eight days and make this a lifestyle. At some point you'll feel confident enough to create your own meal plans built around your favorite meals and recipes (see page 251 for guidance on how to do this).

Don't Let Your Deal Breakers Derail You

We all have certain foods or drinks that we love above all else, and these are often the ones that come to mind the moment someone suggests a diet change. "You mean I'll never be able to have X again?" we ask. Too often, the idea of never having X again becomes a dietary deal breaker—a reason not to change at all.

For this reason, we follow the old saying "Never say never." Sure, if your favorite food is a highly processed, calorie-dense snack, or some form of processed meat, we don't recommend that you include it in your diet regularly. But it's also not worth derailing your entire transition. Turn deal breakers into allies by allowing yourself an occasional indulgence. The key is not to let them become a slippery slope back to old eating habits.

When you think about your favorite foods, ask what exactly it is that you love about them. One thing we've noticed is that they are often connected with meaningful occasions—pizza with buddies, ice cream with grandchildren, waffles at brunch with best friends, pizza on that long-anticipated trip to Italy with your sweetheart. Sometimes these meaningful events—family celebrations, a holiday dinner, or a special date night—are not the worst moments to indulge a little, so long as they don't become the rule. Of course, try to choose the healthiest version of the food available at the time, but more importantly, do it consciously, take responsibility for your choice, and don't tie yourself up in knots of guilt.

Granted, this can be tricky territory. Some find it easier if there's a clear line between what's in and what's out, with no gray area. It's up to you to know yourself and be honest about what will work for you. If you have addictive tendencies, and you know that you find it hard to know when to stop, you might be better off to ignore this strategy and keep things black and white. If you're facing a life-threatening illness, like cancer or heart disease, you may not be able to afford much deviation from a whole foods, plant-based diet. If you crave salty, fatty, or sugary foods, you may find it helpful to leave those out of your diet completely for a period of time until your palate has adapted to the subtler flavors of real food (more on this in chapter 11). However, if you want to make the transition but you're worried about never having that favorite food again, take the *never* out of the equation and see whether it helps you move ahead.

It's far better to change your diet while making room for your deal breaker than not make the change at all. We encourage people to write their deal breakers on a piece of paper and then take them off the table. Don't worry about it anymore. Focus on all the other meals and occasions, and after some time you may be surprised to discover that your deal breaker is not nearly as important as it used to be. In the end, what matters is what you do most of the time, not the small exceptions you might make for a special moment.

Eating Well When Eating Out

Eating a whole foods, plant-based diet at home can be a challenge at first, but once you have your systems in place it will quickly become much easier. The next frontier, for many people, is eating out. It's not always easy to eat well at restaurants, but it can be done, especially if you plan. Here are some tips to navigate meals away from home:

Choose the restaurant. Make sure you have a say in the decision if at all possible. If you've done your homework on local restaurants, you should be able to suggest several options for your dining companions to choose among.

Know your best bets. A traditional American steak house might not be first in line. Asian restaurants in particular often have many plant-based options and are usually happy to make rice and steamed vegetables with oil-free sauces, with a little direction. Mexican restaurants offer rice and beans (but choose whole beans over refried ones, which are often cooked with lard, and soft, not fried, corn tortillas). Add salsa fresca, sliced avocado, and a couple of corn tortillas and you have a satisfying Whole Foodie meal. Try Thai, Indian, or Ethiopian food. If you do visit a meat-oriented restaurant like a steak house or seafood place, see what you can do with salads and vegetable sides (often baked potatoes are available). Or, if you eat animal foods, this might be the time to eat your 10% (or less) portion.

Plan ahead. When possible, look at the menu online before visiting, or give the restaurant a call and ask whether it can accommodate your needs.

Crowd out before you leave the house. If you're not choosing the restaurant—for example, if a friend invites you for a birthday dinner at a place you know has very few options—fill up first with a green smoothie, some leftovers, or a quick and easy whole foods, plant-based meal, then order a salad at the restaurant with balsamic vinegar as dressing. And if you choose to indulge, at least your full stomach will deter you from eating too much.

Be aware of hidden ingredients. This is particularly important if you're trying to eat 100% plant-based foods. You'll want to ask about chicken broth in vegetable soups, lard in beans, butter in rice, and fish stock or fish sauce in many Asian dishes.

Get creative. You may feel uncomfortable asking a chef to create something entirely new for you, but it's OK to get creative with what's already on the menu. You might be surprised how many chefs, when asked nicely, will be happy to help you meet your dietary needs. It is often easier to tell them what you can eat instead of what you can't, so feel free to give a little more guidance if you feel comfortable doing so. Ask for vegetables steamed rather than sautéed. Order a combination of sides and appetizers if there is no plant-based entrée. Be sure to check out the sides that come with the entrées—sometimes these are not listed under "sides," but the waiter will happily bring them if you ask. Or see if there's a sauce on another dish—a marinara, for example—that you could request with steamed veggies or a baked potato. When ordering a salad, ask for dressing on the side or request a bottle of vinegar or a lemon wedge so you can dress it yourself without oil. Soups can sometimes make great sauces.

Don't be afraid to ask! The staff might say no, but even if they do, you've made them better aware of the needs of people like you. Not only are you standing up for your own health, you're also doing a service to others. The more a restaurant gets asked for healthy, plant-based options, the more likely it is to start adding them to the menu.

Do your best. You may not be able to perfectly adhere to your diet outside your own kitchen, but if you don't eat out often, rest easy knowing you've done what you can and you'll do even better the next day when you cook for yourself. If you eat "off the plan" because that was the best you could do, it's not a big deal. But it's important to know yourself and be honest about your motivations. If you feel deprived and choose to eat out as an excuse to satisfy your cravings, while justifying it to yourself as your only option, then you may need to reevaluate how you're approaching the changes you want to make. Maybe you're going too fast. Maybe you're not eating enough. Maybe you need to expand your repertoire and find better ways to satisfy cravings with healthier versions of the foods you love.

Forks on the Road: Whole Foodie Travel Tips

When traveling, as when eating out, planning is essential. Do your homework on the place where you'll stay, local restaurant options, and nearby grocery stores. While it may be tough to eat as well as you do at home, you may be pleasantly surprised by the options available when you know where to look.

If you're choosing a hotel, look for a suites hotel with a small kitchenette in the room. Even just a microwave and fridge make a huge difference. Find a local supermarket when you arrive and stock up on basics, like plant-based milk, oatmeal, fruit, hummus, and ready-cut veggies.

One piece of good news for Whole Foodie travelers is that breakfast on the road is becoming easier, with most hotels and restaurants offering oatmeal and fresh fruit.

Here are some things you might consider taking with you on a trip:

Instant oatmeal with dried fruit and nuts

Whole grain crackers, corn cakes, and brown rice cakes

Trail mix or dried fruit and nuts

Veggies and hummus

Nut butters

Cereal and nondairy milk

Sweet potatoes and hummus (almost all rooms have a microwave and a fridge)

Oil-free chips and salsa or guacamole

Whole wheat bread or pita

Fruit

Prepare Your Family and Friends—But Don't Try to Convert Them!

When we talk to people who are contemplating making a significant diet and lifestyle change, two of the most common concerns we hear are "What will my friends and family think?" and "How will I manage in social situations where everyone else is eating foods I no longer choose to eat?" Food plays a central role in social gatherings, whether it's a Sunday roast dinner with family, burgers with the guys after the game, pizza with the kids, or a weekly brunch with girlfriends. People bond over the shared pleasure of eating, just as humans have done since the dawn of time, and we fear that if we change our eating habits we'll damage those bonds.

These social connections, besides being a source of joy and happiness, are essential to well-being. A meta-analysis of 148 studies shows that the quality and quantity of individuals' social relationships are linked not only to mental health but also to morbidity and mortality.[3] So if you're changing your diet and lifestyle in order to improve your health, the last thing you want that change to do is damage your social connections. It doesn't have to, provided you take care in how you tell your friends about your lifestyle change.

The good news is that plant-based diets are becoming more common and socially acceptable. Your friends might not bat an eyelid when you tell them what you're doing. They may be supportive, surprised, confused, or disbelieving. Worst-case scenario, they may make fun of you or try to change your mind.

Dr. Popper has valuable advice for these moments. "People make it much harder for themselves by thinking they have to convert everyone around them,"[4] she says. Although it's understandable that you might want them to, your family and friends don't have to make the shift with you. You can invite them to join you, but if they don't want to, don't waste your energy being an evangelist. Focus on changing your own habits (and sustaining your newer, healthier ones) and you may naturally inspire others around you to do the same. People don't like feeling pressured or shamed.

Anticipate that some people may feel threatened by your choices, even

Transitioning with Your Family

Changing your own diet and lifestyle is one thing, but where many people balk is at the idea that we have to change our families too. "How am I *ever* going to get my kids to eat kale?" "My kids are picky enough already—they'll just stop eating!" Matt and Alona deal with these questions every day—as parents and as the authors of *Forks over Knives Family: Every Parent's Guide to Raising Healthy, Happy Kids on a Whole-Food, Plant-Based Diet*. Their advice? "At least half the battle is overcoming the false perception that the whole food, plant-based diet is hard and centered on lousy food. The best way to do that is to experience the reality, which is that living this way is all about delicious food shared and eaten together."[5]

Here are a few of their favorite tips from *Forks over Knives Family* to create Whole Foodie homes:

"**Learn together and have fun**—Take the burden off yourself to be the sole purveyor of information about whole food, plant based living by bringing in outside sources and inviting your whole family to join the discussion."[6]

"**Try the gradual approach and be flexible**—Many people successfully implement the lifestyle when they take it slowly.... Success with the gradual approach depends on maintaining an open attitude toward the people in your family you're bringing along."[7]

"**Establish new family habits**—To reinforce the idea that you can implement new, better habits together, introduce some that you all agree to observe—like picking a vegetable or two you'll eat this week."[8]

"**Find a pace that's comfortable for you and your family**—Your goal is to make changes that last a lifetime, so carefully assess and be mindful of what personalities in your house can accommodate. Don't let that hinder your personal goals, if you want to move faster for yourself."[9]

if you're not trying to convert them. Doug Lisle explains that when people hear that someone else is doing something different and "healthier," they experience it as a threat to their status. You may not be criticizing their choices or overtly saying that yours are better, but nevertheless they feel judged (or judge themselves when they see your new choices) and can take your changes personally. Lisle warns that this may manifest itself in their trying to undermine you and tempt you to eat something you've said you don't want. Or it may lead to ridicule, sarcasm, or teasing. Understanding where these behaviors come from won't make them any more fun to deal with, but it will help you to avoid exacerbating them and give you the strength not to succumb to peer pressure.

Get Support

If you live alone, or if your partner or family is not making the transition with you, it is essential that you find support on the journey. Almost every one of the doctors and nutritionists we spoke to while writing this book cited support as a factor that is critical to the success or failure of this kind of transition. It makes all the difference when you have other people to talk to about the changes you're making, the challenges you're facing, the strategies that work for you, and the new favorite foods you're discovering.

You might get this support from a medical professional, a health coach, or a nutritionist. You might also seek out a support group in your area—through your doctor, community wellness program, church group, vegetarian society, or similar resource. You can also try online support groups, of which there are many. Or you could create your own.

If you have like-minded friends who live close by, extend this support into the practical realm by arranging to share dinners on a rotating basis. If you're already cooking for yourself it's simple to cook for a few more, then you receive the benefit of a couple nights off when friends cook for you. You don't have to eat together for this to work—simply prepare the food to be delivered or picked up.

It's important to tell your family and social circle about what you're doing and why, in order to enlist them as allies. Dr. Popper recommends making two requests of family and friends with whom you regularly eat. "First, please don't encourage me to eat these things that are no longer part of my diet. And second, if you see me reaching for them, call me on it."[10]

Recruit Your Doctor to Your Team

Before you begin your transition, talk to your healthcare provider and tell him or her what you are planning to do and why. If you are on any medications to manage a current condition, you should talk about how these might be affected. Switching to a whole foods, plant-based diet can have highly positive

MY WHOLE FOODIE STORY

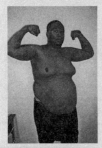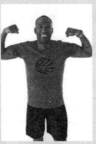

Milan Ross, 45, Mesa, Arizona
"Dad, promise me you'll ride the Harry Potter ride with me!" It was my son's seventh birthday, and my wife and I had taken him to Universal Studios Florida. This was the "most epic ride" he had been waiting for, and I had promised to be by his side. There was just one problem: I weighed well over four hundred pounds, and there was no way I could fit in the seat. As my wife stepped up to take my place, my son cried. It was in that moment that I decided I had to change.

I had a lot of damage to undo—decades of eating a diet of mostly meat, processed foods, fried foods, and sugary drinks. I would regularly consume as many as twelve thousand calories a day, and still not feel satisfied. I never exercised, and I smoked two and a half packs of cigarettes a day. At my heaviest, in my midthirties, I tipped the scales at 518 pounds. I was on meds for high blood pressure, cholesterol, type 2 diabetes, and pain, and every night I had to sleep with a CPAP machine to ensure I didn't stop breathing.

When I returned from Orlando, a colleague at Whole Foods

effects in a short time, so your doctor may need to adjust the dosage of your medications accordingly (especially medications to lower blood pressure and blood sugar) because you could quickly become overmedicated. Request a full blood workup before you begin so you can monitor changes in your cholesterol numbers and other important indicators of success. If your doctor is not supportive of your choice and seems reluctant to work with you on it, you may want to consider finding a more sympathetic ally for your journey. Your doctor does not have to become an expert in plant-based eating, but it is important that he or she is encouraging and does not try to convince you that it is unhealthy. Most importantly, find a doctor who knows how to manage medical

Market, where I'd been working for just over a year, told me about Dr. Stoll's Immersion program and suggested I apply. At first I thought this was just going to be another on-the-job bonus—a free vacation. Instead it turned out to be a transformative event that would alter the trajectory of my entire life.

In just one week, I lost thirty-three pounds and six inches off my waistline, and normalized my blood pressure. In the years since, I have lost well over 225 pounds and twenty-five inches off my waist. I am now off all prescription medications and no longer need a CPAP. My diet has transformed—I still eat a lot of food, but now it's nourishing, healthy, plant-based food. I go to the gym five days a week.

At my heaviest I remember feeling hopeless—condemned to a life of obesity and sickness and early death. I believed I had done so much harm to my body that it could not possibly recover from the damage. I couldn't have been more wrong. I used to have to sit on a chair in my yard to play catch with my son. Now I can play football with him.

To read Milan's day-by-day account of the week that changed his life, check out the book that he coauthored with Dr. Scott Stoll, The Change, *and try their recipes with* The Change Cookbook: Using the Power of Food to Transform Your Body, Your Health, and Your Life.

conditions (if you have any) while also supporting a whole foods, plant-based diet. We have yet to encounter a patient who could not follow a whole foods, plant-based diet because of some medical contraindication. However, once in a while we hear from patients who were told by their doctor that a whole foods, plant-based diet was unsafe for their medical condition. Before conforming to what that doctor says, it would behoove you to get a second opinion from a physician familiar with supporting patients on a whole foods, plant-based diet.

Food Journaling

For some people, keeping a food journal can be useful during the transition to a new dietary pattern. Its purpose is simply to keep you mindful of what you eat or help you and/or your doctor identify areas that may need tweaking if you do not get the health results you think you should. Write down exactly what you ate, including snacks and beverages, and also write down how you feel before, during, and after. How hungry were you before you ate? How satisfied were you afterward? What other feelings do you notice? You may also want to make a note of how you feel at the beginning and end of the day. Are you exhausted when you fall into bed? How well do you sleep? Do you wake feeling rested and energized, or sluggish and groggy? Lastly, note any physical sensations such as digestive trouble, heartburn, or headaches.

Look back over your journal once a week and see what you can learn for the future. If you become stuck with weight loss, you feel constantly hungry, or you have sensitivity to certain foods, your journal can help you decode the problem and come up with a strategy. It may also help you notice when you're comfort eating, and identify unmet needs so you can find better ways to respond. If you binge in the late afternoon, it might be because you're experiencing caffeine withdrawal as you move further away from a morning cup of coffee. You might be trying to satisfy that craving with food, but cutting out the coffee and the resulting withdrawal might be a better solution for some people. If you work with a nutritionist, health coach, or doctor, this journal will be an important tool to help that person help you.

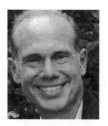

WHOLE FOODIE HERO
Scott Stoll, MD

"Food has the power to prevent, reverse, or suspend most common diseases, as well as influence your relationships, career, charity work, family life, and spirituality. Food is one of the most important foundations of your existence."

Contributions: Dr. Stoll is a physician, educator, and inspirational leader in the plant-based eating movement. He runs total health immersions for plant-based transitions, and he cofounded the Plantrician Project, which works to develop networks of physicians who are aware of the power of plant-based nutrition. His annual International Plant-Based Nutrition Healthcare Conference is a touchstone for the entire movement.

Fun facts: Along with Dr. Caldwell Esselstyn, Dr. Stoll is one of our two Whole Foodie Hero Olympians. Dr. Stoll was on the 1994 American bobsled team. Today he is team physician to the USA bobsled team and regularly works with Olympic athletes.

Read this: *The Change* (with Milan Ross)

Learn more: drscottstoll.com

Keep It Simple!

If you thrive on novelty and love to be creative in the kitchen, by all means entertain yourself with elaborate new meals. But if you're pressed for time, or simply have other priorities, you don't need to become a gourmet chef or eat overly complicated meals to be a happy, healthy Whole Foodie.

When you find something you like, eat it often. We sometimes eat the same meals on weeknights for several weeks until we get bored and then we change it up. We tend to be more creative on weekends. Cycle through your favorites and just try something new when you feel the need for a change. You may decide to eat the same thing for breakfast every day, and rotate through three lunch options and five dinners. If they work for you, that's perfectly fine.

Ease is something we could all use more of in the midst of our busy lives. So don't make your diet overly complicated, especially when it's new. Get the basics right, learn to cook a few meals you love, and eat plenty of them. Don't worry about the minutiae of how this or that food should be eaten. If you worry about whether you should eat kale raw or cooked, or whether potatoes should be boiled or baked, you can find plenty of people online who will argue passionately one way or another. Our advice to you is: just eat whole plant foods! Choose the way it tastes best to you and enjoy it. Once you become accustomed to the whole foods, plant-based lifestyle, you may choose to study the details of creative food preparation techniques but when you're just starting out, keep it simple.

CHAPTER 13

Change Your Plate, Change the World

By John Mackey

"Every time I sit down to eat, I cast my lot: for mercy, against misery; for the oppressed, against the oppressor; and for compassion, against cruelty. There is a lot of suffering in the world, but how much suffering can be addressed with literally no time or effort on our part? We can just stop supporting it, by making different choices."

—*Bruce Friedrich*

For hundreds of pages now, Matt, Alona, and I have made the case that a whole foods, plant-based diet is by far the optimal diet for health, longevity, and overall physical well-being. We have specifically made those arguments based on our understanding of what the very best science says about food and nutrition at this point in history, and I hope that on that basis alone we've convinced you that eating more plants, fewer animals, and fewer highly processed foods makes sense. This has not been a book about the ethics of eating, or how the food we eat might have a beneficial impact on the world around us. However, those are concerns that are close to my own heart, so in this chapter I want to explore those issues and to share some of my personal values and convictions.

As I said in the introduction, I'm a vegan—an ethical vegan. I didn't initially choose this path for my physical health. Don't get me wrong—it's been the best decision I could have possibly made for my own health and well-being, but that was not my initial motivation. I think a vegan diet, if it is based on eating whole foods, can be an extraordinarily healthy diet, far superior to what most Americans are eating today, and research confirms this to be true. Science shows us that vegans who eat whole foods are successful in living long and healthy lives. However, it's quite possible to be an unhealthy junk-food vegan too, so we shouldn't equate veganism with health.

The reason I've not emphasized a vegan diet in these pages is that I don't want to let my ethical beliefs get in the way of the science. And I don't think one needs to be 100% plant-based to eat a very healthy diet. As we've shown, the world's longest-lived cultures eat, on average, a 90% plant-based diet, and there is not sufficient evidence, as far as I can see, that health outcomes differ significantly between 90% and 100%. Some disagree with me on this point, and advocate a 100% vegan diet for health reasons. They may well be correct, but I think the science does not yet justify this position (with the exception of those attempting to reverse chronic disease). Who knows, perhaps one day science will find there are some animal foods, eaten in limited amounts, that are more important than we currently realize for our overall health. Or perhaps science will prove the opposite to be true—that being vegan is more beneficial from a health perspective than we currently appreciate.

Whether one chooses to go 90%, 95%, or 100% plant-based, the Whole Foods Diet outlined in these pages is not just a healthy diet; it is an ethical diet. It will make a tremendous difference in reducing suffering and other unfortunate impacts of animal agriculture. Adopting a plant-based diet, in my mind, means adopting a deeply ethical, caring, and compassionate relationship to the world around us. You may choose to eat some animal foods, but if you do, I hope you will not do so thoughtlessly. And you may also choose to set aside these foods based on your own contemplation of the ethics of doing so.

Our choices, when it comes to eating, have more power than we realize. I'm a businessman and there is nothing I love more than a deal that is truly win-win. Nutrition is one of those rare win-win-win-win situations in

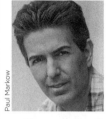

Paul Markow

WHOLE FOODIE HERO
Wayne Pacelle

"If you are part of the old inhumane economic order, get a new business plan or get out of the way. You are already in danger of being too late. Every day there is...less tolerance for self-serving rationalizations for calculated [animal] cruelty. The old ways of thinking are being squeezed into oblivion."

Contributions: As president and CEO of the Humane Society of the United States, Wayne Pacelle has used his position to advocate for animal welfare on multiple fronts. From drafting new legislation to working with businesses like McDonald's and Walmart to improving legal protections for animals, he has been a force of positive change when it comes to transforming our relationship with the animal world.

Fun facts: Pacelle brings his dog, Lilly, to work with him every day, thanks to a pets-in-the-office policy that he instituted when he took over as president of HSUS.

Read this: *The Humane Economy*

Learn more: humanesociety.org

life where what is best for us, healthwise, is also what is best for the world around us, for the animals we share this planet with, for the beauty and health of the natural world, and even, I would humbly suggest, for the care of our self and soul. What we eat is not just personal; it is also political, and of great consequence to the communities in which we live—local, regional, national, and even global.

Compassion for Animals

The ethics of eating animals starts with the sobering reality of the animal farming system that we have today—the industrialized factory farm. When it comes to the way we treat animals as they make their journey through life and onto our plates, the actual killing of them may be the least of our crimes. Anyone who has done even a little research into current methods of meat and dairy production will see the horrific suffering that is inflicted every day on billions of individual animals—pigs, chickens, cows, turkeys— before they make their way to our dinner tables.

Farming today is not the same as it was in an earlier more agrarian society, when we might have had a backyard flock of chickens and a family cow or sow that lived a reasonably good life until the time came to kill and eat them to feed the family. Today farming is a mass-produced outsourced killing machine. In 2015, 9.2 billion livestock animals were killed (along with tens of billions of sea creatures) in the United States alone.[1] Luckily, it does seem that the Western appetite for meat and fish is perhaps topping out, but it is rapidly rising in other parts of the world, along with populations (see graph, page 236).

Whether one decides to eat animals or not, I find the practices of this industry extremely disturbing. That is not to speak ill of any particular business or executives, many of whom are good people trying to meet the needs of consumers worldwide. After all, there is an incessant need to feed more and more people, as meat consumption increases as the world grows richer, and its appetites grow accordingly. You simply can't feed billions of people inexpensive meat every day with the family farms of yesteryear. But slowly, decision by decision, we have built a massive animal-torturing machine and outsourced consumer responsibility to an industrial nightmare. And we have done it with the choices that Americans make every day—to eat meat and to ignore the consequences.

I could easily list some of the inhumane practices that are routinely practiced—from culling (killing) millions of baby chicks to the ugly realities of slaughtering large cows to the squalor of the feedlots—but I will spare you the gory details. Suffice to say they are not pretty, nor do they speak well of human nature. As a famous plant-eater, Paul McCartney, once said, "If slaughterhouses had glass walls, everyone would be a vegetarian."[2]

The animals suffer. They are in pain. They often have short, nasty, and brutish lives. This treatment is something that we need to evolve beyond as a society, not double down on. I suspect that one day we will consider our current treatment of animals to be in the same category as less evolved, more brutal and inhumane practices, like child labor, slavery, genocide, racism, and the oppression of women.

People often ask me, how can you feel this way and still sell meat at Whole Foods Market? I don't have the power to dictate what we sell or what people buy. Like all businesses, Whole Foods Market must respond to the needs and desires of its customers in the marketplace or it will go out of business, as its customers migrate to other stores that will better meet their needs and desires. What I have been able to do is use the platform of Whole Foods Market to raise awareness of the choices we make every day when we buy animal foods. My passion for animal ethics has led me to develop robust animal welfare standards at Whole Foods, the first of their kind in the nation. We do sell meat, fish, and other animal products, but I wanted to make sure that consumers could see where their meals are coming from and how those animals were raised, and encourage the adoption of better standards throughout the industry, creating a "race to the top" for animal welfare. I would love it if Whole Foods were pushed to sell only plant foods because that's what consumers demanded! But until that day comes, I hope Whole Foods will continue to lead the food industry in promoting better forms of animal agriculture.

Despite the ethical challenges that we face in reforming our systems, I remain optimistic that progress can be made, and relatively quickly. Consumers are changing. Despite resistance from established industries, despite many attempts to capture and control the levers of scientific research, and despite the fetishistic elevation of meat in various subcultures, progress is being made. The plant-based movement is growing rapidly. As my friend Wayne Pacelle, executive director of the Humane Society, who has probably done more than anyone to reduce animal suffering in this country, writes in his sobering but highly optimistic book, *The Humane Economy,*

By every measure, life will be better when human
satisfaction and need are no longer built upon the
foundation of animal cruelty. Indefensible practices will
no longer need defending; unnecessary evils will no longer
need excuses. In their place, in market after market, we'll
see the products of human creativity inspired by human
compassion, a combination that can solve any problem
and overcome any wrong...We'll become more alert to
animals, more appreciative of their goodness and their
beauty, and more grateful, as we should be, for how they
fill the world with sounds, colors, and sights, that enrich
every one of us in more ways than we know. [3]

Once we get beyond the painful ethics of the factory farm in its current
form, we come back to the more fundamental question of whether we
should eat animals at all. There is a good reason many deeply ethical men
and women throughout history have chosen to be vegetarian. They did not
want to participate in the killing of animals and the consumption of their
flesh. Indeed, vegetarianism is almost as old as civilization itself. For much of
European history, a near-vegetarian diet was referred to as the Pythagorean
diet, named after one of the most famous vegetarians in history, the mystic
mathematician Pythagoras, who felt that "all life forms should...be treated
as kindred."[4] Plotinus, the Essenes, the Buddha, Virgil, Leonardo da Vinci,
Voltaire, George Bernard Shaw, Albert Schweitzer, Will Durant, Nikola Tesla,
Isaac Newton, Gandhi, even Albert Einstein at the end of his life—the list of
history's famous vegetarians is long and distinguished. And of course, today,
it is an increasingly common choice.

I grew up with beloved family dogs. I own a ranch, which is also home to
several cats, chickens, a donkey, a horse, and countless wild animals. I've come
to know many animals as individual beings with all their quirks, attitudes,
and personalities—not human, but certainly worthy of our respect and
capable of profound relationships. I know they have feelings not dissimilar to
mine. Research has shown again and again that many animals have cognitive

richness, emotional depth, and social complexity. Simply because they are not human, and do not have the same self-reflective qualities that are part of our cognitive repertoire, does not mean that they have no ethical value. Whatever differences exist between human biology, psychology, and sociology and that of many animals, the similarities are far more important. As the English utilitarian philosopher Jeremy Bentham once wrote, the issue is not "can they reason? Can they talk? But, can they suffer?"[5]

Animals experience pain. They clearly suffer—emotionally and physically. Whatever else we might say about plants, there is not really any convincing evidence that they suffer. I think it says something quite interesting about human consciousness that we are able to develop such intimate, heartfelt, and enduring relationships with members of another species. Yet that is hard to square with the reality of the decisions we make around food. Indeed, the many contradictions of what Professor Melanie Joy refers to as human "carnism," the unspoken ideology we use to justify eating meat, are well documented, and (I would suggest) ethically and morally hard to rationalize or defend. Her book title, *Why We Love Dogs, Eat Pigs, and Wear Cows: An Introduction to Carnism*, highlights the issue. Do these distinctions make any sense? By all accounts pigs are extraordinary animals, intelligent and capable of great emotion. Should we eat our dogs? Some cultures do. But in this country that seems abhorrent. There is an unjustified arbitrariness to theses attitudes that speaks to the ill-considered nature of our ethics around animals. In his classic *Animal Liberation*, one of the first books I read on the topic, Peter Singer puts it bluntly:

> To protest about bullfighting in Spain, the eating of dogs in South Korea, or the slaughter of baby seals in Canada while continuing to eat eggs from hens who have spent their lives crammed into cages, or veal from calves who have been deprived of their mothers, their proper diet, and the freedom to lie down with their legs extended, is like denouncing apartheid in South Africa while asking your neighbors not to sell their houses to blacks.[6]

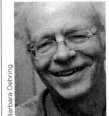

WHOLE FOODIE HERO
Peter Singer, AC

"All the arguments to prove man's superiority cannot shatter this hard fact: in suffering the animals are our equals."

Contributions: Few people in history have made such an impact on the issue of animal suffering as Australian moral philosopher Peter Singer. His book *Animal Liberation*, published in 1975, has become a classic, influencing generations of animal rights activists and ethical vegans.

Fun facts: In 2009, *Time* magazine named Singer one of the hundred most influential people in the world.

Read this: *Animal Liberation*

Learn more: petersinger.info

We don't need to look far afield for ethical reasons not to eat animals. Sometimes we just need to reflect seriously on the inconsistency of our own choices. Whether the decision to abstain from eating animals is born out of a deep love for the animals we personally know, a respect for the beauty and dignity of the animal kingdom, or simply a deep ethical and moral integrity, I do think it represents the better angels of our nature.

Environmental Concerns

I'm an avid hiker. My trail name is "Strider," because I spend so much time walking the paths of this country and many others. It's one of the things I enjoy most. I love the beauty of the natural world, and spending time in that beauty is something I do whenever I can.

While I love my time in nature, and I believe in the conservation of wild places, I don't pretend that there is some original, perfect natural order to the planet that we can preserve as if it were in an eternal museum. Humans have been changing the environment around them in all kinds of ways for thousands of years. Beyond our efforts, the natural world itself is always in a state of flux and change—sometimes subtly, sometimes dramatically. Still, many human impacts on the natural world are significantly, and unnecessarily, harming the rich and diverse ecosystems that sustain so much of the life of this planet—including our own. The recognition of this fact and the desire to mitigate that harm is the essence of environmentalism. And the simple truth is that I don't think there is a single greater act of environmental activism than moving to a plant-based diet.

How many environmentalists appreciate this? How many even acknowledge it? Even if we look beyond the ethics of killing billions of animals a year for our consumption, and focus only on environmental issues, the facts are quite powerful. From climate change to emptying the oceans to land use and forest destruction to habitat loss to water issues to straightforward pollution, our current system of farming, and eating is not doing human health, animal health, or the health of the natural world any favors. It is an inconvenient truth that we cannot ignore any longer.

Climate change is a case in point. I'm certainly not the first one to point out the questionable judgment of those who are passionate about these issues and yet still eat significant amounts of meat. Our appetite for animal products is a major driver of greenhouse gas emissions, and yet the public awareness of this fact is very low.[7] Currently, even low-end estimates suggest that animal agriculture contributes around 18% of global greenhouse emissions, more than the combined exhaust of all transportation emissions.[8] And with the worldwide trend toward consuming more meat and dairy, those emissions are expected to rise by almost 80% over the next few decades.[9]

Growing feed crops for agriculture consumes 56% of the water in the United States.[10] And the global water footprint of feed crops is likely to rise, as wealthier populations of China and India jump on the higher-animal-consumption train. Human dietary appetites are one of the leading causes of species extinction, ocean dead zones, and habitat destruction. Indeed, as animal food consumption increases around the world, not only is this change wreaking havoc on people's health and having extremely negative consequences for the animals themselves (as industrialized factory farms spread everywhere), it is also compromising the sustainability of our global environment.

World Animal Protein Production, 1961–2014

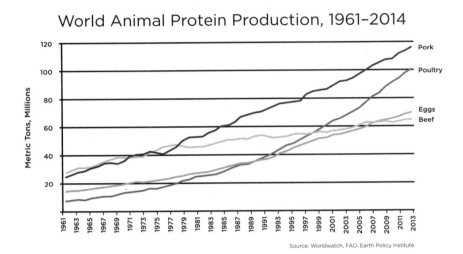

Source: Worldwatch, FAO, Earth Policy Institute.

Reverence for Life

When I was in my thirties, I was introduced to the work and ideas of Albert Schweitzer. I was deeply moved by both his beautiful writing and the way he expressed his philosophy in his own life. He became one of my intellectual and spiritual heroes. His "reverence for life" is something I have long considered a cornerstone of my own approach to living.

Influenced by the Indian concept of *ahimsa*, or nonharming and nonviolence, Schweitzer felt progress was inherently linked to an evolution of our ethics. For him, ethics meant that we have a deep reverence for life and a responsibility toward living things—to enhance them, to affirm them, to avoid needless suffering and death. Schweitzer asks us to consider: How do we live the most compassionate life possible? How do we live a conscious life that minimizes suffering?

There are very few areas in life where we have the chance to reduce suffering so directly and dramatically as in the decision to abstain from consuming animal flesh or other products. I'm not suggesting that somehow we can create a world without suffering or violence. Of course that is impossible. I'm not aiming for an unattainable perfection, or an unreachable state of perfect peace. Suffering is part of life, and definitely part of animal life. Animals suffer and die every day in nature. Many kill for their food. But as conscious and caring human beings, we have the unusual opportunity to not add to that suffering by our own actions. Unlike many animals in nature, we don't *have* to kill other animals to survive. I do think it's an important responsibility—to be conscious of the consequences of our eating choices, to be cognizant of the pain that we may cause these sentient beings whom we may never know or see.

While I don't believe in a perfect world, I do believe in a better world. As never before in our history, more and more people have the freedom to consciously shape our relationship to food and all the consequences that flow from our choices around it. That freedom is also a privilege, and one I hope we will begin to use to create a more conscious society, one that we can be transparently proud of.

The history of the past few hundreds of years of human culture, from one point of view, has been a story of increasing emancipation from various philosophies, theologies, and ideologies that have circumscribed rather than expanded the sphere of human freedom. Why should we stop at the borders of human consciousness? "We must take the final step in expanding the circle of ethics,"[11] writes Singer. I don't know if it's the final step, but I certainly think it is a next step.

To me, reverence for life means that we appreciate the magnificence of life and that we seek to enhance and support it where we can. And it means that we seek to minimize the suffering that we encounter in the world. "By having reverence for life, we enter into a spiritual relationship with the world,"[12] wrote Schweitzer. I agree with him. It is easy for the spiritually sensitive individual to feel overwhelmed by the amount of suffering in the world and to feel incapable of addressing that suffering in any direct and meaningful way. In this arena, however, that is not the case. The choice to abstain from eating animals is not difficult, and it is becoming easier and easier with each passing year. For me it has been one of the most important decisions of my life.

Let me end this chapter by telling a personal story. Back in late 2004, I had the opportunity to meet and take to dinner one of my personal heroes, the great Nobel Prize–winning economist Milton Friedman. My wife and I went to pick up Milton and his wife, Rose, at their home in San Francisco. Milton invited us in for a drink before dinner, and he showed us his home and his Nobel Prize.

While we were chatting in his living room, Milton asked me why I had become a vegan. I told him that I was an ethical vegan and that I wanted to lessen unnecessary animal suffering. I made a challenge to him as well. I told him that I would put forth a brief argument to him and that if he could adequately answer the argument, I would personally stop being a vegan. However, if he couldn't adequately answer the argument, then I expected him to change his own personal diet and become a vegan too. Milton accepted the challenge. There were four parts to the argument:

1. If you eat animals it is absolutely necessary that the animals die. Also, in the United States, more than 99% of the animals that you eat were raised in industrialized factory farms and had lives full of misery and suffering.

2. You don't need to eat animals to have excellent health. Indeed, the science shows that a 100% whole foods, plant-based diet can be one of the healthiest diets you could possibly eat in terms of both health and longevity.

3. The reason we eat animals is that it is how we were raised. It is the result of our family and our culture. Over time we learned to enjoy the taste of animals and it became an accepted part of our personal lifestyle and identity.

4. Can you ethically justify causing the necessary death of animals and the cruelty and inevitable suffering that accompanies it in the industrialized factory farm system just for the pleasure that eating those animals gives to your palate? I cannot justify this ethically myself, so I have chosen to be a vegan. How do you personally justify it?

After I made this argument to Milton he became very quiet for a few minutes as he thought about it. Then he looked at his watch and said that we needed to leave immediately if we weren't going to be late for our dinner reservation at the famous vegetarian restaurant Greens in San Francisco. On the drive over, Milton remained quiet and just occasionally gave me some navigation instructions. Once we arrived we were immediately seated and given our menus. By that time I had decided that Milton wasn't going to try to answer my argument, and I set about studying the menu and figuring out what I wanted to eat. My wife, Deborah, and Milton and Rose did the same thing.

After about a minute of studying his menu Milton then did something that completely astounded and delighted me! He threw his menu down on the table and said, "Rose, I cannot adequately answer John's argument to my own satisfaction. I don't want to cause unnecessary suffering and death to animals just for my own pleasure. From this point forward I'm going to become a vegan!" What happened next was also delightful and funny. Rose Friedman threw her own menu down on the table and said, "Milton, don't be ridiculous! We are ninety-two years old! It is too late for us to become vegans!"

I don't know for sure whether Milton Friedman did change his diet in the last couple years of his life. He was a man of tremendous intellectual integrity, so I would like to think that he did. However, perhaps his wife of sixty-eight years had the final word in the argument and at ninety-two years of age, it really was too late for him to change. Whatever the end to that story may have been, one thing I know for sure is that it isn't too late for you, the reader, to change. You can transform your personal health, as well as lessen the suffering of animals and the degradation of our global environment, by choosing to eat a whole foods, plant-based diet. Matt, Alona, and I have all made this choice ourselves, and we invite you to join us.

PART III

THE 28-DAY
EAT REAL FOOD® PLAN
MEAL PLANS AND
RECIPES

CHAPTER 14

28 Days to Transform Your Health

Welcome to the 28-Day Eat Real Food Plan! We're so happy you've reached this point in the book, and are perhaps considering diving into four full weeks of whole foods, plant-based eating. In this chapter, you'll find:

- **Preparation tips** including a **basic shopping list** (see page 244).
- **Whole Foodie Basics**—quick and easy blueprints to create whole foods, plant-based meals when you're in too much of a hurry to use a recipe (see page 248).
- **How to Use the 28-Day Meal Plan,** including instructions for **batch-cooking** (see page 251) and **making the most of leftovers** (see page 252).
- **The 28-Day Eat Real Food Plan,** which includes instructions for breakfast, lunch, and dinner each day and for batch-cooking each weekend (see page 253).

In the next chapter, you'll find more than thirty delicious, nutritious recipes—from everyday staples to dinner-party delights.

Preparing for Your 28-Day Eat Real Food® Plan

In preparation for your twenty-eight days of eating real food, there are two critical steps to take: clean house (to get rid of the foods you'll no longer eat) and stock up on new, healthy options.

continued on page 246

Whole Foodie Basics Shopping List

✓ **Whole grains**—Brown rice, quinoa, barley, millet, etc. *You can buy these in the bulk section or in bags.*

✓ **Dried beans and lentils**—Black beans, cannellini beans, garbanzo beans, kidney beans, pinto beans, red lentils, brown lentils, French lentils, etc. *You can buy these in the bulk section or in bags.*

✓ **Canned beans** (no added salt)—Black, cannellini, garbanzo, kidney, pinto, etc. *More expensive than dried beans, these are handy to have on hand for when you need a quick meal.*

✓ **Oatmeal**—steel-cut or rolled

✓ **Whole grain pasta**—100% whole wheat, along with brown rice, quinoa, whole spelt, etc.

✓ **Canned tomatoes** (no added salt)

✓ **Oil- and sugar-free marinara sauce**

✓ **Vegetable broth** (low-sodium with no added oil)

✓ **Frozen fruits**—including berries, mangoes, grapes, bananas, and other favorites. *Use these in smoothies, stir them into oatmeal, or eat them right out of the freezer as a snack.*

✓ **Frozen vegetables**—including corn, mixed green veggies, and any other favorites. *Call on these when you have very little time; they are just as health-promoting as fresh veggies.*

✓ **Frozen cooked whole grains**—Look for brown rice or whole grain medleys. *Keep on hand in a pinch—you can defrost them in the microwave, steam, or toss straight into soup.*

✓ **Nuts** (no added oil, salt, or sugar)

✓ **Flax- and/or chia seeds**

✓ **Cold cereals** (no added sugar or refined grains)—such as puffed corn, rice, millet, and kamut

✓ **Condiments**—Look for sugar-free mustard, hot sauce, sriracha, Tabasco, and so on.

✓ **Soy sauce** (low sodium) or Bragg Liquid Aminos

✓ **Vinegars**—Balsamic, apple cider, red wine, etc.

✓ **Fresh fruits**—including berries, bananas, apples, lemon or lime for dressings, and any other favorites. *These are perishable, so buy only what you need for a week.*

- ✓ **Fresh vegetables**—including leafy greens (like spinach, kale, romaine), cruciferous veggies (like broccoli or cauliflower), starchy vegetables (like potatoes or sweet potatoes), other vegetables (like green beans, zucchini, peppers, onions, mushrooms, garlic), and any other favorites. *These are perishable, so buy only what you need for a week.*
- ✓ **Fresh salsa** (oil-free)
- ✓ **Hummus**—We like the Roots and Engine 2 brands, with no added oil.
- ✓ **Tofu**
- ✓ **Tempeh**
- ✓ **Miso**—Start with lighter varieties if you're not accustomed to miso.
- ✓ **Dried fruits**—including dates, raisins, mango, and any other favorites
- ✓ **Unsweetened applesauce**
- ✓ **Nut or soy milk** (unsweetened)—We like the WestSoy brand, specifically the unsweetened plain soy milk.
- ✓ **Frozen veggie burgers**—We like Engine 2 brand, with no added oil. *These are great for a quick meal or snack, and you can heat them in the toaster!*
- ✓ **Corn or whole wheat tortillas**—*You can use these to make easy oil-free chips too (see technique, page 273).*
- ✓ **Whole grain wraps**—We like the Engine 2 and Ezekiel 4:9 brands.
- ✓ **Whole grain pizza crust**—We like Engine 2 brand as well as Nature's Hilights, which is also gluten-free. *Keep them in the freezer for a fast dinner option.*
- ✓ **100% whole grain bread**—We like Dave's Killer Bread Good Seed variety and Ezekial.
- ✓ **Brown rice or corn cakes**—or other whole grain, oil-free crackers (try Mary's Gone Crackers for gluten-free varieties)
- ✓ **Nut butter** (no added oil or sugar)
- ✓ **Herbs and Spices**—Basil, oregano, thyme, bay leaves, onion powder, garlic powder, ginger, black pepper, nutmeg, cinnamon, paprika, cayenne, crushed red pepper, turmeric

continued from page 243

STEP ONE. Clean House!

When you begin a transition to a whole foods, plant-based lifestyle and decide to remove certain foods from your diet, it's wise to remove them from your kitchen as well. If those foods are easily accessible, they will be that much more appealing. Lani Muelrath, who has written a helpful and detailed guide to this diet transition, *The Plant-Based Journey*, writes, "Whatever it is that compels you to the cupboard, it's going to call to you, no matter how nicely you ask it not to. If it is a preoccupational hazard, you are probably better off not having it in the house for now."[1]

Equip Your Kitchen: Helpful Tools

Blender and/or food processor—If you enjoy smoothies, a really good high-powered blender makes a huge difference. You'll also find it useful for making dressings, sauces, and soups. The two best high-powered blenders we know of are Vitamix and Blendtec, and while they are significant investments, they are well worth it. A food processor can also be useful for making spreads like hummus, and immersion blenders are great for soups.

Nonstick pans—For cooking without oil, a good nonstick pan makes all the difference. Choose ceramic titanium or cast iron and avoid the Teflon-coated ones, which have potential toxicities associated with them. If you don't want to buy a whole set right away, start with a large, high-sided skillet or wok—you can use this for stir-fries, scrambles, sauces, and even soups.

A good knife and cutting board—Whole Foodie eating involves a lot of vegetables, so you'll appreciate having a nice sharp knife for preparation.

Pressure cooker—If you have limited time for meal preparation, using a pressure cooker is a wonderful way to speed up the process of cooking beans, soups, stews, and many other foods.

Rice cooker or slow cooker—These surprisingly affordable tools take the guesswork out of cooking grains, and also allow you to slow-cook things like soups, stews, and even oatmeal overnight.

Start by removing all highly processed foods, especially those containing lots of sugar, white flour, oil, and salt. You don't want to make it harder for yourself by keeping your pantry stocked with cookies or chips and your fridge full of soda or ice cream. Get rid of processed meats, such as hot dogs, lunch meats, and bacon as well. You will need space for all the wonderful fresh produce and wholesome foods you'll stock up on. Take time to clean house and prepare your kitchen both practically and symbolically for your new lifestyle. If you feel bad about throwing out food, consider donating it to a local food bank or community kitchen.

If you live with family or roommates who are not making the transition with you, it may not be possible to remove all the foods you will no longer eat. Perhaps you can rearrange so those items live only in a certain cupboard or on a certain shelf. Family members may also be willing to support you by keeping certain foods out of the house, even if they continue to eat them elsewhere.

STEP TWO. Stock Up

Once you've cleaned your fridge and pantry, you're ready to go shopping. You're going to want to have plenty of delicious healthy foods readily available in your home! Your recipes will help you know what you need to buy for specific meals,

Know Your Numbers

There are many measures of health, and we want you to see progress in those areas that are meaningful to you. In addition to feeling better and potentially seeing disease symptoms improve, you may also see improvement in some of the following health markers: blood pressure, heart rate, weight, waist circumference, body mass index (BMI), blood cholesterol (total cholesterol, triglycerides, LDL, HDL), and diabetes markers (e.g., hemoglobin A1c). Before you begin following a whole foods, plant-based diet, discuss your medical history with your personal doctor along with which markers would make sense to measure before and after you begin your personal program (see page 222 for more on recruiting your doctor to your team).

but there are also basics that are good to keep on hand. On pages 244–245 you'll find our shopping list, and over time you'll develop your own lists of favorites.

Whole Foodie Basics

Chef-created recipes are wonderful for introducing you to new flavors and fresh ways to prepare delicious, nutritious meals. But we all have days when there is simply no time to reach for a recipe book, and we just want to throw together a quick meal with ingredients from the fridge, the freezer, or the pantry. That's where the Whole Foodie Basics come in. You don't need a recipe to create these meals—just follow the basic blueprints and create your own meals using whatever ingredients you have on hand. Any of these options will provide a simple, satisfying meal that won't take you long to prepare.

Note: Suggested quantities are per serving; adapt as needed to feel satisfied.

Whole Foodie Breakfast Bowl

Oatmeal or cold cereal is a hearty base for combinations of fruits and some nuts.

> **Base—oatmeal (cooked, see technique page 265) or cold cereal (unsweetened) with soy or other nondairy milk**
>
> **Toppings—favorite fruits, fresh or frozen**
>
> **Optional—1 small handful of chopped nuts or dried fruit**

Whole Foodie Wrap

Perfect for lunch on the run, a whole grain wrap with hearty bean spread and lots of fresh veggies can provide a satisfying and portable meal.

> **Whole grain wrap—whole wheat, brown rice, or other**
>
> **Bean spread—hummus (see recipe, page 281), black bean spread, white bean spread, or other**
>
> **A couple handfuls of salad greens—romaine, baby spinach, arugula, spring mix, or other**
>
> **Other raw veggies—try grated carrots or zucchini, sliced cucumbers, radishes, tomatoes, or peppers, or anything else you have in your fridge**

A condiment—whole grain mustard, salsa, sriracha sauce, Oil-Free
Herb Pesto (see recipe, page 299), relish

Optional: to make a fuller meal, add cold cooked grains such as brown
rice or quinoa, or sliced avocado.

Whole Foodie Salad

Salads don't have to be appetizers—add whole grains and beans,
along with greens and plenty of raw or cooked veggies for a full meal.

A big bowl of greens—romaine, baby spinach, arugula, kale,
spring mix, or other

1 cup of raw or cooked veggies—steamed broccoli or cauliflower,
crunchy snow peas, radishes, cucumbers, peppers, or any other
favorites

½ to 1 cup beans (precooked or canned, rinsed)black, pinto,
cannellini, garbanzo, or other

½ to 1 cup whole grains (precooked or frozen)—brown rice, quinoa,
barley, or whichever grain you have batch-cooked this week

Oil-free dressing (see formula, page 279)

Whole Foodie Bowl

The variations on a meal in a bowl are endless (see pages
286–287 for some of our favorites). Here's a simple formula for
making your own Whole Foodie bowls.

1 to 2 cups steamed or raw greens—spinach, kale, romaine, or other

1 cup whole grains (precooked or frozen)—brown rice, quinoa,
barley, or whichever grain you have batch-cooked this week

1 to 2 cups steamed veggies—broccoli, cauliflower, green beans,
zucchini, or other

1 cup beans (precooked or canned, rinsed)—warm these with
veggie broth, a little soy sauce or Bragg Liquid Aminos, and your
favorite herbs and spices. Add enough liquid to become a sauce.

To assemble, put greens in a bowl, pile grains and steamed veggies on top,
then pour beans and sauce over the whole bowl and enjoy!

Optional: You can also experiment with making oil-free sauces for your bowls (like No-Oil Marinara, page 283, or a variety of nut- and seed-based sauces you can easily make in your high-speed blender).

Whole Foodie Smoothie

Sometimes you need to eat breakfast on the run, and that's when a smoothie is a quick choice. For those trying to lose weight, eating breakfast (e.g., oatmeal and fruit) over drinking breakfast (e.g., smoothie) may help you reach your goals more efficiently. Find two of our favorite smoothie recipes on page 267, but when you want to create your own, follow this blueprint:

1 banana

1 cup of other fruit (fresh or frozen)—berries, apple, mango, pear, or other

A couple big handfuls of raw greens—kale, spinach, romaine, or other

1 small handful of nuts—or a tablespoon of chia seeds or ground flaxseeds

Water or unsweetened nondairy milk of your choice—1 to 2 cups, depending on how thick you like your smoothie

Blend all ingredients and enjoy

Animal Foods on the 28-Day Eat Real Food® Plan

This 28-Day Eat Real Food Plan can be 100% plant-based, or you can choose to eat some animal foods (10% or less of your calories). Some of our recommended recipes include an animal food option; others can easily be adapted. For example, you might add some grilled chicken or fish to a stir-fry or salad, add a little cheese as a topping to a pasta dish or a salad, or add an egg at breakfast.

To keep your animal foods below 10% of your calories, treat them as a condiment and eat no more than once a day (see page 167 for sample quantities) or save them for a special meal once or twice a week in larger servings.

How to Use the 28-Day Meal Plan

We've designed the 28-Day Eat Real Food Plan using the recipes found in chapter 15 of this book. You can follow it exactly, or mix and match to suit your preferences. If you're pressed for time, you can always fall back on one of our Whole Foodie Basics (see page 248).

Remember, we want you to eat enough and feel satisfied, so if any of our suggested meals doesn't fill you up, add extra fruit or veggies, have some hearty whole grain bread with your soup, or start your meal with a big salad that includes grains and beans.

As you gain confidence in Whole Foodie eating and cooking, use this template to create your own meal plans based on your favorites. Here are the principles that underlie our plan, which you can also use when you begin to create your own.

Plan a week of meals at a time. If you work Monday to Friday, you might do your planning Friday evening or Saturday morning, including making a shopping list, so you can use some time on the weekend to shop and prepare. If you use our plan, look over the recipes we suggest and make shopping lists accordingly.

Make your ingredients multitask. Especially if you're cooking for only one or two people, it makes sense to plan several meals that use similar ingredients. That way you won't end up with half-used bags of produce, bunches of herbs, cans of beans, or jars of condiments.

Batch-cook. If you are able to set aside a couple hours once a week for what's known as batch-cooking—preparing staples in large quantities for use throughout the week or to be frozen in serving-size bags for reheating—you can save a lot of time on the day-to-day meals. Many people like to do this on Sunday afternoon or evening. You'll see that the 28-Day Eat Real Food Plan includes a weekly batch-cooking session, with tasks such as:

- Cook a big pot of whole grains
- Cook a big pot of beans (or use canned beans if you prefer)
- Cook a big pot of soup that you can reheat for a couple lunches
- Bake potatoes or sweet potatoes
- Make sandwich or wrap fillings (hummus, baked tofu, etc.)

You may also want to:

- Steam a big batch of mixed vegetables—they'll keep for a few days and you can add them cold to salads
- Wash the fruits and vegetables
- Wash and dry the greens
- Cut snack-size sticks of carrot, celery, and peppers
- Blend up a jar of no-oil salad dressing (see formula, page 279)
- Make homemade nut milk (see technique, page 266)

If you don't have time to do all this, or just don't feel like spending the time in the kitchen, consider buying ready-washed, cut, or prepared versions of these foods at many markets.

Love your leftovers! Even when it's not your weekly batch-cooking session, get in the habit of making more than you'll need. Our plan often repurposes leftovers from dinner for lunch the next day, and we'll tell you when you need to cook extra. You can also cook extra and freeze in portion-size containers for nights when you just don't have time to do more than defrost, warm, and serve.

The 28-Day Eat Real Food® Plan

A Note about Servings: Most of our recipes are designed for four people (unless stated otherwise), but these are simply guidelines, and we want to encourage you to cook and eat enough that you feel satisfied, and to adapt the recipes accordingly. In our batch-cooking instructions, we tell you how many servings you need to make per person so you can calculate the appropriate quantity. As you become familiar with cooking this way, you'll learn how much to prepare. And it's never a problem if you make too much—just eat as leftovers or freeze for the future.

WEEK 1

ON THE WEEKEND	MONDAY	TUESDAY	WEDNESDAY
Cook brown rice (see technique, page 286)—Cook enough for at least five servings per person.	**BREAKFAST** Whole Foodie Breakfast Bowl with oatmeal or cold cereal, fresh fruit *See page 248 for basic recipe and ideas.*	**BREAKFAST** Whole Foodie Breakfast Bowl with oatmeal or cold cereal, fresh fruit *See page 248 for basic recipe and ideas.*	**BREAKFAST** Whole Foodie Breakfast Bowl with oatmeal or cold cereal, fresh fruit *See page 248 for basic recipe and ideas.*
Bake tofu (see technique, page 285)—Make enough for at least two servings per person. Cut half in cubes *(for topping)* and the rest in slices *(for sandwich fillings).*	**OR** Smoothie *See recipe, page 250; eat extra fresh fruit if still hungry.*	**OR** Smoothie *See recipe, page 250; eat extra fresh fruit if still hungry.*	**OR** Smoothie *See recipe, page 250; eat extra fresh fruit if still hungry.*
Make hummus (see recipe, page 281)—Make enough for at least two servings per person. *(If you don't have time, buy oil-free hummus.)*	**LUNCH** Whole Foodie Wrap with hummus and veggies Use the hummus you made (or an oil-free brand) on a whole grain wrap, and add lots of greens and veggies. *See recipe, page 248.*	**LUNCH** Hearty Split Pea and Spinach Soup, whole grain bread You prepared this on the weekend—heat, stir in the baby spinach, and enjoy.	**LUNCH** Baked tofu sandwich with avocado and sprouts Use the baked tofu you made on the weekend as the filling for a satisfying sandwich, together with mustard, fresh greens or sprouts, and sliced tomatoes.
Make Hearty Split Pea and Spinach Soup (see recipe, page 270)—Make enough for at least two servings per person. Tip: don't add the spinach yet—toss it in when you reheat so it's fresh and green.	**DINNER** Romantic Rice Bowl with chicken or tofu *See recipe, page 286.* Use the rice and baked tofu cubes you made on the weekend, or add chicken if you prefer.	**DINNER** Penne Puttanesca with Roasted Red Pepper Sauce over whole wheat pasta, green salad *See recipe, page 297.*	**DINNER** Mushroom Stroganoff with brown rice, green salad *See recipe, page 291.* You can steam or microwave the brown rice you cooked on the weekend. NOTE: Make twice as much as you need—you'll have this again for lunch tomorrow.

THURSDAY	FRIDAY	SATURDAY	SUNDAY
BREAKFAST Whole Foodie Breakfast Bowl with oatmeal or cold cereal, fresh fruit *See page 248 for basic recipe and ideas.* **OR** Smoothie *See recipe, page 250; eat extra fresh fruit if still hungry.*	**BREAKFAST** Whole Foodie Breakfast Bowl with oatmeal or cold cereal, fresh fruit *See page 248 for basic recipe and ideas.* **OR** Smoothie *See recipe, page 250; eat extra fresh fruit if still hungry.*	**BREAKFAST** Veggie and Tofu Scramble *See recipe, page 268.*	**BREAKFAST** Whole Wheat Blueberry Pancakes *See recipe, page 269.*
LUNCH Mushroom Stroganoff with brown rice leftovers, green salad	**LUNCH** Whole Foodie Wrap with hummus and herb pesto Use the hummus you made on the weekend or an oil-free brand; add the herb pesto from last night as a condiment and lots of fresh veggies.	**LUNCH** Pineapple-Ginger Rice Bowl and Kale Waldorf Salad leftovers Use the leftovers from last night's dinner.	**LUNCH** Garden Picnic Pasta Salad with Veggies, Herbs, and Orange-Miso Tahini Dressing Enjoy last night's pasta again for lunch today.
DINNER Hearty Split Pea and Spinach Soup, Pita Pizza with Herb Pesto and Green Veggies Use the rest of the soup you prepared on the weekend. *See Pita Pizza recipe, page 298.* NOTE: Make extra herb pesto to use in a lunch wrap tomorrow.	**DINNER** Pineapple-Ginger Rice Bowl with Edamame, Kale Waldorf Salad *See recipes, pages 280 and 288.* Make extra to have for lunch over the weekend.	**DINNER** Garden Picnic Pasta Salad with Veggies, Herbs, and Orange-Miso Tahini Dressing, steamed greens *See recipes, pages 301 and 302.* Make extra—this pasta salad is served cold and will make a perfect lunch for tomorrow.	**DINNER** Baked sweet potatoes with Cashew Sour Cream, steamed veggies, salad *See recipe, page 284.* NOTE: You'll bake sweet potatoes as part of your batch-cooking for next week, so make enough for dinner as well.

WEEK 2

ON THE WEEKEND	MONDAY	TUESDAY	WEDNESDAY
Bake sweet potatoes—Cook enough for at least three servings per person. (Cook a couple extra if you'd like to try making our Sweet Potato Chocolate Mousse on page 305 this week!) Cook quinoa (see technique, page 287)—Cook enough for at least three servings per person. Cook pinto beans (see technique, page 288)—Cook enough for at least three servings per person. (If you don't have time, use canned beans.) Make Not-Tuna Salad (see recipe, page 278)—Make enough for at least two servings per person. Make Fresh Salsa (see recipe, page 284)—Make enough for at least two servings per person. (This is very quick to make, but if you don't have time, buy oil-free salsa.)	**BREAKFAST** Whole Foodie Breakfast Bowl with oatmeal or cold cereal, fresh fruit *See page 248 for basic recipe and ideas.* **OR** Smoothie *See recipe, page 250; eat extra fresh fruit if still hungry.*	**BREAKFAST** Whole Foodie Breakfast Bowl with oatmeal or cold cereal, fresh fruit *See page 248 for basic recipe and ideas.* Try taking some of your baked sweet potatoes and mashing them in with oatmeal and cinnamon. **OR** Smoothie *See recipe, page 250; eat extra fresh fruit if still hungry.*	**BREAKFAST** Whole Foodie Breakfast Bowl with oatmeal or cold cereal, fresh fruit *See page 248 for basic recipe and ideas.* **OR** Smoothie *See recipe, page 250; eat extra fresh fruit if still hungry.*
	LUNCH Whole Foodie Wrap with Not-Tuna Salad Use the salad you made on the weekend as a filling for your wrap, along with fresh greens or veggies in your fridge.	**LUNCH** Sesame Peanut Noodles Enjoy last night's dinner as a chilled noodle salad for lunch.	**LUNCH** Not-Tuna Salad sandwich, Cream of Cauliflower and White Bean Soup with Garlic Croutons *See recipe, page 275.*
	DINNER Cream of Cauliflower and White Bean Soup with Garlic Croutons *See recipe, page 275. Make extra!* Sesame Peanut Noodles *See recipe, page 295. Make extra for lunch tomorrow—these are great cold.*	**DINNER** Mighty Bowl of Goodness *See recipe, page 287.* Use precooked quinoa for this nourishing meal in a bowl.	**DINNER** Refried Beans and Avocado Soft Tacos *See recipe, page 300.* Use the pinto beans you cooked on the weekend. Make extra refried beans to use for your lunch burrito tomorrow. Use your fresh salsa too.

THURSDAY	FRIDAY	SATURDAY	SUNDAY
BREAKFAST Whole Foodie Breakfast Bowl with oatmeal or cold cereal, fresh fruit *See page 248 for basic recipe and ideas.* **OR** Smoothie *See recipe, page 250; eat extra fresh fruit if still hungry.*	**BREAKFAST** Whole Foodie Breakfast Bowl with oatmeal or cold cereal, fresh fruit *See page 248 for basic recipe and ideas.* **OR** Smoothie *See recipe, page 250; eat extra fresh fruit if still hungry.*	**BREAKFAST** Veggie and Tofu Scramble *See recipe, page 268.*	**BREAKFAST** Whole Wheat Blueberry Pancakes *See recipe, page 269.*
LUNCH Whole Foodie burrito Use the extra refried beans from last night, along with cooked quinoa, salsa, avocado, and lettuce to make a delicious burrito with your favorite whole grain wrap.	**LUNCH** Whole Foodie Salad with quinoa and pinto beans Use the last of your precooked quinoa and beans to fill out a big salad.	**LUNCH** Whole Foodie Wrap with hummus, greens, and veggies *See recipe, page 248.*	**LUNCH** Smoky Bean and Root Veg Chili *See recipe, page 276.* You'll be batch-cooking this hearty chili for next week, but get an early start and you can eat it for lunch as well.
DINNER Mashed Sweet Potatoes, Kale Waldorf Salad *See recipe, page 280.* Use some of your baked sweet potatoes.	**DINNER** Pita Pizza with Herb Pesto and Green Veggies *See recipe, page 298.* Try different veggies than when you made this last night. Make lots of extra herb pesto—you'll use this tomorrow for dinner.	**DINNER** Whole grain spaghetti with herb pesto and roasted veggies Use half of the extra herb pesto you made last night as a sauce for the pasta. Use the rest to coat veggies (whatever you have in the fridge) and roast in the oven until they start to brown.	**DINNER** Baked potatoes with Cashew-Chive Sour Cream, salad You'll be baking potatoes as part of your batch-cooking for next week, so make enough for dinner as well! *See recipe, page 284.*

WEEK 3

ON THE WEEKEND	MONDAY	TUESDAY	WEDNESDAY
Bake potatoes— Make enough for at least two servings per person. **Make White Bean Hummus** (see recipe, page 281; substitute cannellini beans for garbanzos)—Make enough for at least two servings per person. **Cook barley** (or brown rice if gluten-free; see technique, page 286)—Make enough for at least two servings per person. **Make Smoky Bean and Root Veg Chili** (see recipe, page 276)—Make enough for at least three servings per person. **Make No-Oil Marinara** (see recipe, page 283)—Make enough for at least one serving per person plus extra to freeze. *(If you don't have time, buy oil-free marinara—look for the Engine 2 brand or the Whole Foods Market 365 brand.)*	**BREAKFAST** Whole Foodie Breakfast Bowl with oatmeal or cold cereal, fresh fruit *See page 248 for basic recipe and ideas.* **OR** Smoothie *See recipe, page 250; eat extra fresh fruit if still hungry.*	**BREAKFAST** Whole Foodie Breakfast Bowl with oatmeal or cold cereal, fresh fruit *See page 248 for basic recipe and ideas.* **OR** Smoothie *See recipe, page 250; eat extra fresh fruit if still hungry.*	**BREAKFAST** Whole Foodie Breakfast Bowl with oatmeal or cold cereal, fresh fruit *See page 248 for basic recipe and ideas.* **OR** Smoothie *See recipe, page 250; eat extra fresh fruit if still hungry.*
	LUNCH Whole Foodie Wrap with white bean hummus and veggies *See recipe, page 248; use the hummus you made on the weekend.*	**LUNCH** Tempeh Curry with Sweet Potatoes and Green Beans leftovers	**LUNCH** Whole grain sandwich with white bean hummus, roasted red peppers, and avocado
	DINNER Tempeh Curry with Sweet Potatoes and Green Beans, brown rice, salad *See recipe, page 292.* Make extra curry so you can have it for lunch tomorrow.	**DINNER** Whole Foodie Bowl with pasta and No-Oil Marinara Sauce *See recipe, page 283.* Get creative with whatever veggies are in your fridge— steam them and add to whole grain pasta to make a simple bowl topped with the marinara sauce you made on the weekend.	**DINNER** Smoky Bean and Root Veg Chili over barley (or brown rice if gluten-free), green salad Use the chili and barley you made on the weekend.

THURSDAY	FRIDAY	SATURDAY	SUNDAY
BREAKFAST	**BREAKFAST**	**BREAKFAST**	**BREAKFAST**
Whole Foodie Breakfast Bowl with oatmeal or cold cereal, fresh fruit	Whole Foodie Breakfast Bowl with oatmeal or cold cereal, fresh fruit	Veggie and Tofu Scramble	Whole Wheat Blueberry Pancakes
See page 248 for basic recipe and ideas.	*See page 248 for basic recipe and ideas.*	*See recipe, page 268.*	*See recipe, page 269.*
OR	**OR**		
Smoothie	Smoothie		
See recipe, page 250; eat extra fresh fruit if still hungry.	*See recipe, page 250; eat extra fresh fruit if still hungry.*		
LUNCH	**LUNCH**	**LUNCH**	**LUNCH**
Smoky Bean and Root Veg Chili leftovers, green salad	Mushroom Stroganoff leftovers, barley, green salad	Asian Wild Rice and Kale Salad leftovers	Whole Foodie Salad with Indian-Spiced Veggie Burger leftovers
			Slice the extra burgers you made last night to top a hearty salad with cold whole grains and lots of veggies.
DINNER	**DINNER**	**DINNER**	**DINNER**
Mushroom Stroganoff with mashed potatoes, Kale Waldorf Salad	Asian Wild Rice and Kale Salad with Toasted Seeds and Miso-Citrus Dressing	Indian-Spiced Veggie Burgers, sweet potato No-Oil Fries	Coconut Corn Chowder, whole grain bread, steamed veggies
See recipes, pages 280 and 291.	*See recipe, page 280.*	*See recipes, pages 293 and 294.*	*See recipe, page 273.*
Make extra for lunch tomorrow!	Make extra for lunch tomorrow!		You'll be batch-cooking this delicious soup to eat next week, so make enough for dinner tonight as well. Serve with hearty whole grain bread and steamed veggies.
Remember the delicious Mushroom Stroganoff with brown rice from week one? Now try it as a topping for mashed potatoes (make these with baked potatoes, mashed with a little nondairy milk).			

WEEK 4

ON THE WEEKEND	MONDAY	TUESDAY	WEDNESDAY
Bake tempeh (see technique, page 285)—Make enough for at least two servings per person. **Cook black beans** (see technique, page 288)—Make enough for at least four servings per person. **Cook brown rice** (see technique, page 286)—Make enough for at least three servings per person. **Make Coconut Corn Chowder** (see recipe, page 273)—Make enough for at least two servings per person. **Make Fresh Salsa** (see recipe, page 284)—Make enough for at least three servings per person. *(If you don't have time, buy oil-free salsa.)*	**BREAKFAST** Whole Foodie Breakfast Bowl with oatmeal or cold cereal, fresh fruit *See page 248 for basic recipe and ideas.* **OR** Smoothie *See recipe, page 250; eat extra fresh fruit if still hungry.*	**BREAKFAST** Whole Foodie Breakfast Bowl with oatmeal or cold cereal, fresh fruit *See page 248 for basic recipe and ideas.* **OR** Smoothie *See recipe, page 250; eat extra fresh fruit if still hungry.*	**BREAKFAST** Whole Foodie Breakfast Bowl with oatmeal or cold cereal, fresh fruit *See page 248 for basic recipe and ideas.* **OR** Smoothie *See recipe, page 250; eat extra fresh fruit if still hungry*
	LUNCH Whole Foodie Wrap with baked tempeh, hummus, greens, and veggies *See recipe, page 248.*	**LUNCH** Black Bean Salad with Avocado-Lime Dressing *See recipe, page 278.* This is a quick salad to make using precooked black beans and frozen corn. Serve on a bed of greens.	**LUNCH** Jhap Chae Stir-Fry with noodles Reheat the leftovers from Monday night's dinner for lunch.
	DINNER Jhap Chae Stir-Fry with noodles *See recipe, page 296.* Make extra so you can eat this for lunch on Wednesday.	**DINNER** Pineapple-Ginger Rice Bowl with Edamame *See recipe, page 288.*	**DINNER** Austin Taco Bowl *See recipe, page 289.* Use your precooked black beans and brown rice to make this quickly and easily. Make extra so you can use leftovers for a burrito lunch tomorrow.

THURSDAY	FRIDAY	SATURDAY	SUNDAY
BREAKFAST Whole Foodie Breakfast Bowl with oatmeal or cold cereal, fresh fruit *See page 248 for basic recipe and ideas.* **OR** Smoothie *See recipe, page 250; eat extra fresh fruit if still hungry*	**BREAKFAST** Whole Foodie Breakfast Bowl with oatmeal or cold cereal, fresh fruit *See page 248 for basic recipe and ideas.* **OR** Smoothie *See recipe, page 250; eat extra fresh fruit if still hungry*	**BREAKFAST** Veggie and Tofu Scramble *See recipe, page 268.*	**BREAKFAST** Whole Wheat Blueberry Pancakes *See recipe, page 269.*
LUNCH Whole Foodie burrito The leftovers from last night's taco bowl make an easy burrito filling for lunch.	**LUNCH** Whole grain tempeh BLT sandwich Use your baked tempeh in place of bacon and add lettuce and tomato.	**LUNCH** Spicy Tortilla Soup with Black Beans Enjoy the leftovers from last night's soup for lunch.	**LUNCH** Penne Puttanesca with Roasted Red Pepper Sauce leftovers, green salad
DINNER Coconut Corn Chowder, whole grain bread, salad Use the last of the soup you made on the weekend for this simple, satisfying dinner.	**DINNER** Spicy Tortilla Soup with Black Beans *See recipe, page 271.* Use the last of your black beans for this fun Friday night soup.	**DINNER** Penne Puttanesca with Roasted Red Pepper Sauce, green salad *See recipe, page 297.* Remember this delicious zesty pasta from week one? Make enough so you can enjoy it for lunch tomorrow as well.	**DINNER** Garden-Stuffed Potato Cacciatore with a big Whole Foodie Salad *See recipes, pages 249 and 302.* You might plan to batch-cook baked potatoes for next week today while you're making this dinner.

CHAPTER 15

Whole Foodie Recipes

BREAKFASTS

Oatmeal Fruit Shake

How to Cook Oatmeal

How to Make Nut Milk

Pumpkin Pie Smoothie

Breakfast Green Machine Smoothie

Veggie and Tofu Scramble

Whole Wheat Blueberry Pancakes

SOUPS

Hearty Split Pea and Spinach Soup

How to Sauté without Oil

Spicy Tortilla Soup with Black Beans

Mexican Spice Blend

Coconut Corn Chowder

How to Make No-Oil Tortilla Chips

Cream of Cauliflower and White Bean Soup with Garlic Croutons

Smoky Bean and Root Veg Chili

SALADS

Not-Tuna Salad

Black Bean Salad with Avocado-Lime Dressing

How to Make No-Oil Salad Dressing

Kale Waldorf Salad

Asian Wild Rice and Kale Salad with Toasted Seeds and
  Miso-Citrus Dressing

SPREADS, SAUCES, AND SANDWICH FILLINGS

Simple No-Oil Hummus

Spicy BBQ Tahini Sauce

How to Make White Balsamic Glaze

No-Oil Marinara Sauce

Fresh Salsa

Cashew Sour Cream

How to Make Baked Tofu or Tempeh

WHOLE BOWL MEALS

Romantic Rice Bowl

How to Cook Rice

Mighty Bowl of Goodness

How to Cook Quinoa

Pineapple-Ginger Rice Bowl with Edamame

How to Cook Beans

Austin Taco Bowl

Red Pepper Pico

Avocado-Jalapeño Crème

ENTRÉES

Mushroom Stroganoff

Tempeh Curry with Sweet Potatoes and Green Beans

Indian-Spiced Veggie Burgers

How to Make No-Oil Fries

Sesame Peanut Noodles

Jhap Chae Stir-Fry

Penne Puttanesca with Roasted Red Pepper Sauce

Pita Pizza with Herb Pesto and Green Veggies

Oil-Free Herb Pesto

Refried Bean and Avocado Soft Tacos

Garden Picnic Pasta Salad with Veggies, Herbs, and
    Orange-Miso Tahini Dressing

Garden-Stuffed Potato Cacciatore

DESSERTS AND SWEETS

Oatmeal-Raisin Cookies

Sweet Potato Chocolate Mousse

Raspberry Nice Cream

BREAKFASTS

Oatmeal Fruit Shake

Created by Derek Sarno

Serves 2

Make too much oatmeal? This is a healthful way to use the extra for a quick, nutritious smoothie with flavorful options.

- 1 cup oatmeal, already prepared and cooled (see basic technique, below)
- 1 apple, cored and roughly chopped

continued

How to Cook Oatmeal

Oatmeal is a wonderful nutritious breakfast that lends itself to many variations of toppings and flavors. You can try rolled oats, which cook quickly and have a soft texture, or steel-cut oats, which take a little longer and produce a more chewy oatmeal. Oatmeal can be made with water or your favorite nondairy milk (although this option increases calorie density). You can also cook oatmeal overnight—simply bring to a boil, then turn off the heat and cover. In the morning just reheat and serve.

Rolled oats: Use 1 cup dry oats to 2 cups water or nondairy milk. Bring to boil, then simmer, stirring occasionally, until oats are tender and consistency is as thick as you like (5 to 12 minutes).

Steel-cut oats: Use 1 cup dry oats to 2 to 3 cups water or nondairy milk. Bring to boil, then simmer, stirring occasionally, until oats are tender and consistency is as thick as you like (10 to 30 minutes depending on brand). If you have a rice cooker, try soaking the oats overnight in the rice cooker, then turning it on in the morning—your oatmeal will be ready in about 20 minutes.

Topping ideas: Stir in frozen berries and a few nuts or a small handful of raisins, top with fresh fruit, stir in cooked sweet potato and cinnamon, make it savory with tamari, spinach, and chopped nuts—get creative!

1 banana, peeled and halved

1 cup baby spinach

2 cups coconut water

2 cups ice

½ teaspoon ground cinnamon

1 teaspoon pure vanilla extract

Add all ingredients to blender.

Blend from low to high for several minutes until smooth.

Recipe note: Play with different versions by using a nondairy milk instead of coconut water for added creaminess or by using different fruits, such as berries or mango (frozen or fresh). Adjust thickness by adding less or more liquid.

Per serving: 270 calories, 1.5g total fat, 0g saturated fat, 0mg cholesterol, 65mg sodium, 58g total carbohydrate (7g dietary fiber, 28g sugar, 0g added sugars), 5g protein, 2mg iron

How to Make Nut Milk

1 cup nuts makes about 2¾ cups

Making nut milk is easy—just allow time to soak the nuts. Try almonds, walnuts, cashews, or hazelnuts.

Soak the nuts for at least 10 hours in cold water.

Combine nuts and 3 cups fresh water in a blender and blend until very smooth.

Strain through a double thickness of cheesecloth, a fine-mesh strainer, or a nut-milk bag (optional).

Note: Unless you use the nut milk for coffee or tea, it doesn't need to be strained and you can keep all that healthy fiber. Just shake or stir the pitcher every time you use it.

Refrigerate in an airtight container up to three days.

Pumpkin Pie Smoothie

Serves 2

This delectable, healthful smoothie is packed with nutrients. Top each serving with ground flaxseeds or a pinch of nutmeg if you like.

- 1 **cup pumpkin puree**
- 1 **large ripe banana**
- 1 **cup unsweetened soy milk or almond milk**
- 2 **pitted dates**
- ½ **teaspoon pure vanilla extract**
- 1¼ **teaspoons pumpkin pie spice**
- 5 **ice cubes**
  Ground flaxseeds, to taste (optional)
  Pinch of nutmeg (optional)

Combine all ingredients in a blender and blend until smooth.

Per serving: 150 calories, 2.5g total fat, 0g saturated fat, 0mg cholesterol, 65mg sodium, 30g total carbohydrate (4g dietary fiber, 17g sugar, 0g added sugars), 5g protein, 1mg iron

Breakfast Green Machine Smoothie

Created by Chad Sarno

Serves 2

This vegetable- and fruit-packed smoothie is a nutritious meal on the go. With the addition of matcha green tea powder, this smoothie will give a kick of energy to start your day off right.

- 1 **cup peeled and chopped cucumber (1 medium cucumber)**
- 2 **or 3 leaves green kale**
- ½ **cup baby spinach**
- 1 **banana, peeled**
- ½ **cup frozen mango**
- 3 **tablespoons hemp hearts (buy these in most natural foods stores)**
- 1 **teaspoon matcha (find this green tea powder in the tea section of most natural foods stores)**

continued

1 **cup nondairy milk of your choice, unsweetened**

Combine all ingredients in a blender and blend on high until smooth.

Per serving: 210 calories, 8g total fat, 1g saturated fat, 0mg cholesterol, 120mg sodium, 29g total carbohydrate (3g dietary fiber, 18g sugar, 0g added sugars), 8g protein, 3mg iron

Veggie and Tofu Scramble

Serves 4

This vegan veggie-packed alternative to scrambled eggs makes a terrific breakfast, lunch, or dinner. Finely chopping vegetables in a food processor saves time, and this step can be done the night before if mornings are hectic. Serve it with whole grain tortillas and your favorite hot sauce if you like.

2 **cups lightly packed spinach leaves**

1 **large tomato, quartered**

½ **red or yellow bell pepper, quartered**

½ **red onion, quartered**

3 **cloves garlic**

1 **(14-ounce) package firm tofu, well drained***

⅛ **teaspoon fine sea salt**

*To drain, remove from packaging, wrap in paper towels, and gently press.

In a food processor, combine spinach, tomato, bell pepper, onion, and garlic, and pulse until finely chopped (or chop by hand). This mixture can be covered and refrigerated up to one day.

Put vegetable mixture in a large skillet and bring to a simmer over medium-high heat. Crumble in tofu and sprinkle with salt. Cook, stirring and breaking up any large chunks of tofu, until most of the liquid has evaporated, about 8 minutes. Serve warm.

Per serving: 120 calories (60 from fat), 7g total fat, 1g saturated fat, 0mg cholesterol, 100mg sodium, 7g total carbohydrate (2g dietary fiber, 2g sugar, 0g added sugars), 12g protein, 2.7mg iron

Whole Wheat Blueberry Pancakes
Serves 4

These whole wheat pancakes are studded with warm blueberries and make a healthy morning treat. Freeze pancakes in stacks of three for breakfast later in the week.

- 2 **cups whole wheat pastry flour**
- 2 **teaspoons baking powder**
- 1 **teaspoon ground cinnamon**
- ¼ **teaspoon fine sea salt**
- 1 **cup unsweetened plain almond milk, soy milk, or rice milk**
- ¼ **cup unsweetened applesauce**
- 1 **teaspoon pure vanilla extract**
- 1¼ **cups fresh or frozen blueberries**

In a large bowl, whisk together flour, baking powder, cinnamon, and salt. In a separate medium bowl, whisk together almond milk, ¼ to ½ cup water (or additional almond milk), applesauce, and vanilla until blended. Pour milk mixture into flour mixture and stir until evenly combined. Set batter aside to rest 10 minutes (batter will be very thick).

Heat a cast-iron griddle or nonstick skillet over medium heat until hot. Stir blueberries into batter. Ladle about ¼ cup batter onto the griddle and cook about 2 minutes or until bottoms are golden. Flip and cook 1 to 2 minutes longer, until pancakes are cooked through.

Per serving (about 3 pancakes): 260 calories (15 from fat), 2g total fat, 0g saturated fat, 0mg cholesterol, 350mg sodium, 52g total carbohydrate (10g dietary fiber, 7g sugar, 0g added sugars), 9g protein, 3mg iron

SOUPS

Hearty Split Pea and Spinach Soup

Created by Derek Sarno

Serves 4 to 6

There is something so nurturing about a warm bowl of soup in your hands with your favorite whole grain seeded bread. This comforting split pea soup is a one pot meal that's perfect for cold days.

- 1 cup diced white onion
- ½ cup diced carrot
- ½ cup diced celery
- 1 cup diced red russet potato
- 4 cloves garlic, minced
- 1 tablespoon minced fresh thyme
- 7 to 8 cups low-sodium vegetable broth (to taste)
- 1½ cups dry green split peas, soaked overnight*
- ¼ cup parsley, lightly packed and chopped, plus more for garnish
- 2 tablespoons fresh lemon juice
- 1 teaspoon ground black pepper
- 4 ounces baby spinach
- 1 lemon, cut into wedges for garnish

*If peas didn't soak, double cooking time (see directions below for details).

Place soup pot on medium to high heat. When pot is heated, add the onion and dry-sauté (see technique, page 271) until onion begins to stick and get slightly translucent. Add the carrot, celery, potato, garlic, and thyme; stir well, allowing to sauté an additional 2 minutes. Add about ¼ cup of the vegetable broth to deglaze the pan if needed.

Add split peas and vegetable broth. Bring to a simmer and allow to cook on low to medium about 20 to 25 minutes. *(Note: If peas did not soak in advance, double this time.)*

How to Sauté without Oil

Cooking without oil may be new to you, but it's not hard—and it's an easy way to make meals that much healthier.

For onions: Place sauté pan on medium to high heat. When pot is heated, add the onions and dry-sauté them, stirring frequently until they begin to stick, you begin to see some coloration on the bottom of the pan, and the onions begin to turn slightly translucent. Add about 2 to 3 tablespoons of vegetable stock (or water) to deglaze the pan and caramelize the onions to start your dish.

For other veggies: Place sauté pan on medium to high heat, and add a little vegetable stock or water to steam-fry veggies.

Add the parsley, lemon juice, pepper, and a bit more broth if needed to thin. Allow to cook 5 to 8 additional minutes.

Turn off heat and stir in spinach. The spinach will steam and wilt in the heat of the soup as you add it.

Garnish with fresh parsley and lemon wedges.

Stir and serve with a slice of your favorite seeded whole grain bread.

Recipe note: This can also be made in a slow cooker set on low for 6 to 8 hours.

Per serving: 290 calories, 1g total fat, 0g saturated fat, 0mg cholesterol, 260mg sodium, 56g total carbohydrate (17g dietary fiber, 12g sugar, 0g added sugars), 18g protein, 4mg iron

Spicy Tortilla Soup with Black Beans
Serves 8

This simple, spicy soup is great for parties. Create a build-your-own-soup bar with avocado, Cashew Sour Cream (see recipe, page 284), chopped lettuce, red onion, and loads of fresh herbs, then let guests create their own delicious bowls.

4   corn tortillas

1   large yellow onion, peeled and diced (about 1 cup)

1   jalapeño pepper, seeded and diced

2   tablespoons Mexican Spice Blend (see recipe, below)

Zest and juice of 1 lime

2   (28-ounce) cans no-salt-added diced tomatoes (or 4 pounds fresh, chopped)

¼   cup chopped fresh cilantro

1   (15-ounce) can no-salt-added black beans, drained and rinsed, for garnish

1   avocado, diced, for garnish

Preheat the oven to 350°F. Place tortillas in a single layer on a rimmed baking sheet. Cook tortillas about 10 minutes, flipping to opposite sides halfway through. Remove from oven when chiplike. Break into bite-size pieces.

Heat a large soup pot over high heat. Add onion, jalapeño, Mexican Spice Blend, and lime zest. Cook until fragrant and onion starts to soften, about 3 minutes. Add water as needed to avoid burning. Add diced tomatoes

Mexican Spice Blend

Makes about 6 tablespoons

Blend together these flavorful spices to elevate any dish, from simple rice and beans or tofu tacos to creamy squash soup. Store in an airtight container.

2   tablespoons paprika

2   tablespoons no-salt-added chili powder

1½ teaspoons onion powder

1½ teaspoons garlic powder

1½ teaspoons ground cumin

1½ teaspoons ground black pepper

¼   teaspoon cayenne or ground chipotle pepper (optional)

and 2 cups water. Bring to a boil, reduce heat to a gentle simmer, and cover. Continue to simmer, 15 to 20 minutes. Puree soup with an upright or immersion blender. Add lime juice and cilantro. Serve with no-oil baked tortilla chips (see technique, below), black beans, and avocado.

Per serving (about 1 cup): 170 calories (40 from fat), 4.5g total fat, 0.5g saturated fat, 0mg cholesterol, 30mg sodium, 27g total carbohydrate (7g dietary fiber, 8g sugar, 0g added sugars), 6g protein, 1mg iron

Coconut Corn Chowder

Created by Derek Sarno

Serves 6

Hearty, fun, and delicious! This is one of our all-time favorites.

- 3 medium russet potatoes, peeled and cut into 1-inch cubes
- 5 or 6 cloves garlic
- 1 cup diced white onion
- 1 tablespoon minced garlic
- 2 tablespoons minced ginger
- 1 teaspoon ground black pepper
- 1 teaspoon crushed red pepper flakes
- 1 bay leaf
- 2 pounds frozen or fresh corn off the cob
- 1 (13.5-ounce) can coconut milk
- Juice of 2 limes
- ¼ cup fresh torn mint leaves plus extra whole mint leaves for garnish
- 1 teaspoon fine sea salt

How to Make No-Oil Tortilla Chips

Most tortilla chips are laden with oil and salt, but you can easily make a healthier version at home! Cut whole grain tortillas in wedges, sprinkle with paprika or cayenne (if you like them spicy), and bake in a 350°F oven until crispy.

Add potatoes and whole garlic cloves to a medium-size pot with enough water to cover. Bring to a boil and cook until tender and a fork can slide through them. Drain, rinse, and save cooking water aside, equivalent to 6 cups.

On stove top, warm a large pot on medium-high heat. When pot is heated, add the onion and dry-sauté (see technique, page 271), stirring frequently until onion begins to stick slightly and you begin to see some coloration on the bottom of the pan, roughly 1 to 2 minutes. Add minced garlic, ginger, and black and red peppers and stir for another minute.

Add water/potato broth (left over from cooking potatoes), bay leaf, and 1 pound of the corn. Bring to a slow boil. Once it begins to boil, lower heat to medium low and allow to simmer.

Separately, in a blender, add the second pound of corn, 1 cup of the cooked potato, and the coconut milk, and blend into a creamy consistency (add a little extra water only if needed to loosen so it blends evenly).

Slowly add this creamy corn mixture to the pot, stirring to mix well with the other ingredients. Add the remaining cooked diced potatoes and allow mixture to slowly come back to a simmer, stirring often.

Right before serving, add lime juice and salt, and stir in torn mint. Garnish with the extra fresh mint sprigs; additional chili peppers are optional.

Variations: This versatile recipe lends itself to creative variations. Basil or Thai basil is a nice addition with the mint and as a garnish. For spice lovers, add fresh Thai chiles or jalapeño, also good for garnishing for those special occasions. For a thick and savory oatmeal, whisk in 1 cup of rinsed oats at the same time you add water. For a festive style, have condiments like fresh bean sprouts, cilantro, mint, basil, and a variety of veggies as topping options.

Per serving: 370 calories, 15g total fat, 12g saturated fat, 0mg cholesterol, 420mg sodium, 60g total carbohydrate (6g dietary fiber, 8g sugar, 0g added sugars), 8g protein, 4mg iron

Cream of Cauliflower and White Bean Soup with Garlic Croutons

Created by Chad Sarno

Serves 4 to 6

The combination of creamy cauliflower and cannellini beans is the best prescription for a cold day. Pair this flavorful soup with crunchy garlic croutons for a hearty meal on its own or as a delicious start to multiple courses.

SOUP

- 2 cups diced white onion
- ¼ cup chopped garlic
- 7 cups low-sodium vegetable broth
- 4 cups cauliflower florets
- ½ cup peeled and cubed white Japanese sweet potato
- 1 (15-ounce) can white cannellini beans, strained and rinsed well
- 2 tablespoons nutritional yeast
- ¼ teaspoon ground white pepper
- 1½ tablespoons onion granules
- 1½ tablespoons garlic granules
  Sea salt to taste

CROUTONS

- 4 slices whole grain bread, cut into large cubes
- 1 tablespoon garlic granules
- ½ tablespoon onion granules
- ¼ teaspoon ground black pepper
  Splash of low-sodium vegetable broth

Place soup pot on medium to high heat. When pot is heated, add the onion and dry-sauté until onion begins to stick and get slightly translucent (see technique, page 271). Add the garlic and stir well, allowing to sauté an additional 2 minutes. Add about ¼ cup of the vegetable stock to deglaze the pan, stirring well.

Reduce heat to medium. Add the remaining ingredients and bring to a simmer, allowing it to simmer about 12 minutes. Turn off heat.

Take pot off heat and, using an immersion blender, blend the soup until smooth. Alternatively, carefully pour into a blender and blend until smooth, then return to the pot.

Place the pot on low heat and continue to cook 5 to 8 minutes, allowing the soup to reduce slightly. Season with sea salt to taste.

To prepare the croutons: Preheat oven to 350°F. In a mixing bowl, toss the cubed bread with the spices and a splash of vegetable broth. The vegetable broth will help the spices stick.

Place on sheet pan lined with parchment paper and bake 4 to 6 minutes or until crisp. Remove and use as croutons for this soup or salads.

Per serving (soup and croutons): 230 calories, 2g total fat, 0g saturated fat, 0mg cholesterol, 440mg sodium, 39g total carbohydrate (6g dietary fiber, 12g sugar, 0g added sugars), 11g protein, 2mg iron

Smoky Bean and Root Veg Chili

Created by Derek Sarno

Serves 4 to 6

This is an ideal recipe for a slow cooker. You can set it and forget it for a few hours. The longer and more slowly it's cooked, the more flavor develops. If you do not have a slow cooker, prepare it on the stovetop in a large pot. There should be plenty for leftovers. Serve with brown rice, barley, farro, or other whole grain on the side.

- 2 (14-ounce) cans kidney beans (no salt added), strained
- 2 (14-ounce) cans pinto beans (no salt added), strained
- 1 (28-ounce) can diced tomatoes (no salt added)
- 1 (26-ounce) can strained tomatoes
- 1 (7-ounce) can tomato paste
- ½ cup dates, pasted (soaked in hot water for one hour and smashed into a paste)
- 1 good-size sweet potato, peeled and diced medium

  2 large carrots, cut in ½-inch half moons

  1 large turnip, diced

  1 medium onion, diced

  4 tablespoons chili powder

  4 tablespoons ground cumin

  1 tablespoon granulated garlic

  1 tablespoon granulated onion

  1 tablespoon ground black pepper

  1 teaspoon coarse sea salt (optional)

  1 teaspoon smoked paprika

  2 bay leaves

In slow cooker: Add all ingredients, stir to incorporate, and cook 4 to 6 hours on high or 6 to 8 hours on low.

On stovetop: Add all ingredients, stir to incorporate, and cook on medium-low heat for several hours, stirring frequently to avoid burning and sticking to the bottom. If you have a large Dutch oven, place in oven at 300°F and cook 3 hours at 325°F, stirring every 30 minutes.

Serve with a whole grain such as brown rice and condiments (see notes below).

Recipe notes and options: This recipe lends itself to a variety of garnishes and assorted toppings. Here are some ideas:

  ¼ cup thinly sliced jalapeños

  1 cup diced red onion

  ½ cup fresh cilantro leaves for garnish

  1 cup Cashew Sour Cream (see recipe, page 284)

  ½ cup black olives, diced

  2 avocados, diced

  ½ cup diced bell peppers (assorted colors for vibrancy)

Per serving (without garnish): 400 calories, 2.5g total fat, 0g saturated fat, 0mg cholesterol, 320mg sodium, 79g total carbohydrate (10g dietary fiber, 26g sugar, 0g added sugars), 18g protein, 5mg iron

SALADS

Not-Tuna Salad

Makes 3 cups

Enjoy the flavor and texture of tuna salad with this vegetarian mixture of garbanzo beans (also known as chickpeas), apples, and pecans. Perfect for sandwiches or wraps, or as a spread on crackers.

- 1 (15-ounce) can no-salt-added garbanzo beans, rinsed and drained
- ½ apple, cored and chopped
- ¼ cup finely chopped celery
- ¼ cup chopped pecans
- 2 tablespoons dill relish
- 2 tablespoons finely chopped red onion
- 2 tablespoons chopped fresh dill
- 2 tablespoons fresh lemon juice
- 1 teaspoon kelp granules
- Ground black pepper to taste

Pulse the garbanzo beans in a food processor until coarsely chopped. Transfer to a medium bowl and add apple, celery, pecans, relish, red onion, dill, lemon juice, and kelp granules. Stir until well combined. Season with pepper and chill until ready to serve.

Per serving (½ cup): 90 calories, 4.5g total fat, 0g saturated fat, 0mg cholesterol, 55mg sodium, 11g total carbohydrate (3g dietary fiber, 3g sugar, 0g added sugars), 3g protein, 0mg iron

Black Bean Salad with Avocado-Lime Dressing

Serves 4

This colorful salad features a quick dressing made from creamy avocado, tangy lime juice, and zesty cilantro.

- 1 ripe avocado, mashed
- ¼ cup chopped fresh cilantro

How to Make No-Oil Salad Dressing

Nuts and fruits can make for creamy, juicy, and flavorful salad dressings without any extracted oils. Plus you get the health benefits of nutrient-dense foods. Save money by using your imagination and what's in your pantry to come up with new flavor combinations, and skip the store-bought dressings, which aren't as healthy or as tasty.

⅓ **cup chopped nuts, such as walnuts, cashews, almonds, or pecans**

½ **cup chopped fresh fruit, such as plums, peaches, blueberries, or strawberries**

¼ **cup unsweetened soy milk or nut milk**

1 tablespoon lemon or lime juice (or vinegar)

Puree all ingredients in a food processor or high-powered blender until smooth.

2 tablespoons lime juice

2 (15-ounce) cans no-salt-added black beans, rinsed and drained

4 cups shredded romaine lettuce

1 cup grape tomatoes, halved

1 cup corn kernels, fresh or thawed if frozen

1 small red bell pepper, chopped

½ cup toasted pumpkin seeds

In a large bowl, whisk together avocado, cilantro, and lime juice until blended. Add beans, lettuce, tomatoes, corn, pepper, and pumpkin seeds, and toss until evenly coated.

Per serving: 400 calories, 17g total fat, 2.5g saturated fat, 0mg cholesterol, 30mg sodium, 49g total carbohydrate (17g dietary fiber, 4g sugar, 0g added sugars), 19g protein, 2mg iron

Kale Waldorf Salad

Serves 4 to 6

This variation on the classic Waldorf salad uses kale instead of lettuce and adds apple and walnuts to the dressing for a creamy consistency without the typical mayonnaise base.

- 4 cups packed finely chopped kale, preferably dinosaur kale
- 1 large red apple, such as Fuji or Honeycrisp, chopped
- 3 large stalks celery, thinly sliced
- ½ cup toasted and chopped walnuts
- ¼ cup plus 2 tablespoons raisins
- 2 tablespoons Dijon mustard
- 1 tablespoon red wine vinegar
- ⅛ teaspoon fine sea salt

Place kale in a large bowl. Add half the apple along with celery, ¼ cup walnuts (keeping ¼ cup for the dressing), and ¼ cup raisins (keeping 2 tablespoons for the dressing).

Put remaining apple in a blender along with remaining ¼ cup walnuts, remaining 2 tablespoons raisins, mustard, 2 tablespoons water, vinegar, and salt. Puree until well combined and slightly thick, adding water if needed to thin. Pour dressing over salad and toss to combine.

Per serving: 130 calories (60 from fat), 7g total fat, 0.5g saturated fat, 0mg cholesterol, 120mg sodium, 16g total carbohydrate (3g dietary fiber, 11g sugar), 2g protein, 0.7mg iron

Asian Wild Rice and Kale Salad with Toasted Seeds and Miso-Citrus Dressing

Created by Chad Sarno

Serves 4

In this Asia-inspired salad, the nuttiness of the wild rice is complemented by the toasted seeds, shredded kale, and sweet acidic dressing with a kick of ginger.

- 3 cups cooked wild rice

  3 tablespoons sliced green onion

  ¼ cup shredded carrot

  2 cups stemmed and shredded kale

  3 tablespoons chopped fresh cilantro

  ¼ cups 100% orange juice

  1 tablespoon unseasoned rice vinegar

  2½ tablespoons white miso

  1 tablespoon finely minced ginger

  1 clove garlic, finely minced

  3 tablespoons dry-toasted sesame seeds

After wild rice is cooked and cooled, hand-mix in the green onion, carrot, kale, and cilantro, and set aside.

In a small bowl, whisk the orange juice, vinegar, miso, ginger, and garlic well until smooth.

Mix the sauce thoroughly with the rice mixture.

Garnish with sesame seeds and serve.

Per serving: 210 calories, 4g total fat, 0g saturated fat, 0mg cholesterol, 330mg sodium, 36g total carbohydrate (3g dietary fiber, 5g sugar, 1g added sugars), 8g protein, 2mg iron

SPREADS, SAUCES, AND SANDWICH FILLINGS

Simple No-Oil Hummus

Serves 6

This homemade hummus is made without the traditional olive oil and is a delicious dip, perfect for entertaining or as a snack. Pair with lightly toasted pita bread, crisp veggies, stuffed grape leaves, and a selection of olives. Cannellini or Great Northern beans can be substituted for the garbanzo beans.

- 2 **cloves garlic**
- 1 **(15-ounce) can no-salt-added garbanzo beans, rinsed and drained**
- 3 **tablespoons lemon juice**
- 2 **tablespoons tahini (sesame paste)**
- ½ **teaspoon ground cumin**
- ½ **teaspoon reduced-sodium tamari**
- ¼ **teaspoon ground coriander**

  Cayenne pepper to taste
- 2 **tablespoons finely chopped fresh parsley**

Put garlic in a food processor and pulse to roughly chop. Add garbanzos, ¼ cup water, lemon juice, tahini, cumin, tamari, coriander, and a pinch of cayenne, and process until creamy and smooth. Transfer to a bowl, cover, and chill for at least 1 hour.

Before serving, let hummus come to room temperature. Stir in parsley.

Per serving: 80 calories, 3.5g total fat, 0g saturated fat, 0mg cholesterol, 25mg sodium, 10g total carbohydrate (2g dietary fiber, 1g sugar, 0g added sugars), 4g protein, 0mg iron

Spicy BBQ Tahini Sauce

Makes about 1½ cups

This delicious earthy, spicy sauce can be used to top your Whole Foodie Bowls, steamed vegetables, baked potatoes, and more.

How to Make White Balsamic Glaze

This simple vinegar syrup is wonderful for drizzling over roasted or steamed veggies.

Pour 2 cups white balsamic vinegar into a small saucepan. Place on medium heat. When it starts to simmer, lower to low-medium heat and continue to reduce until the vinegar becomes thicker and reduced to about ⅓ to ½ cup. (Be sure to put a vent on during this process; the aroma is strong but so worth the sweet acidity of the syrup.)

½ cup tahini

⅓ cup vinegar-based Louisiana-style hot sauce

1 tablespoon tomato paste

1 tablespoon nutritional yeast

1 teaspoon ground cumin

1 teaspoon chili powder

½ teaspoon smoked paprika

½ teaspoon coarse sea salt

½ teaspoon ground black pepper

Add all ingredients to a blender or bowl with ⅓ cup water and whisk together until smooth.

Per serving (about 2 tablespoons): 100 calories, 8g total fat, 1g saturated fat, 0mg cholesterol, 210mg sodium, 4g total carbohydrate (0g dietary fiber, 0g sugar, 0g added sugars), 3g protein, 1mg iron

No-Oil Marinara Sauce

Makes about 3 cups

Use this simple marinara sauce as a topping for your favorite whole grain pasta or for steamed veggies.

½ cup reduced-sodium vegetable broth

1 cup finely chopped white onion

4 cloves garlic, finely chopped

⅛ teaspoon crushed red pepper flakes (optional)

2 tablespoons no-salt-added tomato paste

2 (15-ounce) cans no-salt-added chopped tomatoes

1 tablespoon balsamic vinegar

2 tablespoons thinly sliced fresh basil

1 tablespoon finely chopped fresh oregano

¼ teaspoon fine sea salt

   Freshly ground black pepper

In a large skillet over medium-high heat, bring broth to a simmer. Add onion, garlic, and crushed red pepper and cook until onion is translucent, about 5 minutes. Add tomato paste and cook 1 minute, stirring constantly. Reduce heat to medium, stir in tomatoes, and cook about 15 minutes to blend flavors, stirring occasionally to make sure mixture doesn't stick to the pan. Remove from heat and stir in vinegar, basil, oregano, salt, and pepper. Serve warm or chill until ready to serve.

Per serving (about ¼ cup): 25 calories (0 from fat), 0g total fat, 0g saturated fat, 0mg cholesterol, 95mg sodium, 4g total carbohydrate (1g dietary fiber, 3g sugar), 1g protein, 0.7mg iron

Fresh Salsa

Makes about 2 cups

Salsa has lots of advantages: It seems indulgent, but it's actually a healthy choice because it's fat-free and loaded with flavorful vegetables. It's inexpensive, especially when the ingredients are homegrown or in season. It's versatile because you can make it hotter with more peppers or sweeter with fruit. And it's easy!

- 2 cups chopped tomatoes (or a combination of tomatoes and fresh peaches, nectarines, mangoes, or grapes)
- ⅓ cup chopped yellow or white onion
- 2 tablespoons chopped fresh cilantro
- 2 tablespoons lime juice
- 1 to 2 jalapeño or serrano peppers, stemmed, seeded, and finely chopped
- ¼ teaspoon fine sea salt (optional)

Put all ingredients in a bowl, toss well, and serve chilled or at room temperature.

Per serving (about ½ cup): 25 calories (0 from fat), 0g total fat, 0g saturated fat, 0mg cholesterol, 5mg sodium, 6g total carbohydrate (1g dietary fiber, 3g sugar), 1g protein, 0.3mg iron

Cashew Sour Cream

Makes about 1¼ cups

This simple vegan sour cream is wonderfully rich and tasty. Try it with chopped salads in place of mayonnaise, with anything Mexican, or on its own as a dip for vegetables or crackers.

1   cup raw cashews

2   teaspoons cider vinegar

1   teaspoon lemon juice

⅛   teaspoon fine sea salt

Place cashews in a cup or small bowl and cover by about half an inch with boiling water. Let soak 30 minutes. Drain cashews and place in a blender with vinegar, lemon juice, salt, and about ¼ cup water. Blend until very smooth, adding more water as required to puree the mixture.

Variations: Use lime juice instead of lemon juice and add jalapeño, to taste, for a spicy Mexican sour cream. Add chopped fresh chives or dill to make a delicious topping for baked potatoes.

Per serving (¼ cup): 150 calories, 12g total fat, 2g saturated fat, 0mg cholesterol, 60mg sodium, 8g total carbohydrate (1g dietary fiber, 2g sugar, 0g added sugars), 5g protein, 1mg iron

How to Make Baked Tofu or Tempeh

Savory baked tofu or tempeh can be used as a sandwich filling or added to salads or bowl meals. Try this simple marinade or experiment with adding different herbs and spices.

Makes enough marinade for a 1-pound block of tofu or tempeh

¼   cup low-sodium soy sauce

½   cup balsamic vinegar

2   dates

1   tablespoon Dijon mustard

Preheat the oven to 350°F. Combine all the marinade ingredients in a blender and blend until smooth. Drain tofu and gently press with a paper towel to remove water. Cut tofu or tempeh into cubes (for salads or bowls) or slices (for sandwiches). Toss in the marinade, cover, and leave to sit for at least half an hour. Spread on a baking sheet and bake 15 to 20 minutes.

WHOLE BOWL MEALS

Romantic Rice Bowl

Serves 2

It doesn't have to be Valentine's Day for you to share this "rice bowl built for two" from a large decorative bowl with two pairs of chopsticks.

- ¾ cup low-sodium chicken or vegetable broth
- ⅔ cup uncooked brown rice
- ¼ pound chicken tenderloins or 4 ounces tofu, cubed
- 2 cups broccoli florets
- 2 carrots, thinly sliced
- ½ red bell pepper, thinly sliced
- ½ avocado, thinly sliced
- 1 sheet toasted nori, cut or torn into small pieces
- ¼ cup 100% orange juice
- ½ teaspoon barley miso

Combine broth, ⅔ cup water, rice, and chicken (if using) in a medium pot and bring to a boil. Reduce heat to medium-low, cover, and simmer until rice is almost tender, about 35 minutes.

Scatter broccoli and carrots over rice mixture, cover, and continue to cook until vegetables are tender, 6 to 8 minutes more. Transfer broccoli and

How to Cook Rice

Use 1 cup rice to 2 cups water. Put rice and water into a small pot and bring to a boil over medium-high heat. Reduce heat to medium-low, cover pot, and simmer just until liquid is completely absorbed and rice is tender, about 40 minutes. No peeking until then; valuable steam escapes. Set covered pot off the heat 10 minutes, then uncover and fluff rice with a fork.

For perfect rice every time, you might consider investing in a rice cooker.

carrots to a plate, then shred chicken or add tofu, stirring it into the rice. Spoon rice and chicken into a large bowl and attractively arrange broccoli, carrots, pepper, avocado, and nori on top. In a small bowl, whisk together orange juice and miso; drizzle over bowl, or serve on the side for dipping.

Per serving: 290 calories (80 from fat), 9g total fat, 1.5g saturated fat, 35mg cholesterol, 210mg sodium, 34g total carbohydrate (8g dietary fiber, 8g sugar, 3g added sugar), 20g protein, 1.8mg iron

Mighty Bowl of Goodness
Serves 4

We predict this colorful one-dish meal will become a new favorite.

- 1 **cup quinoa**
- 1 **cup sprouted green lentils or sprouted mung beans**
- 1 **bunch kale, stemmed, chopped, and steamed, or 1 head broccoli, cut into florets and steamed**
- 16 **ounces grilled tofu, chicken, or salmon (optional)**
- 1 **avocado, cut into wedges**

FOR SERVING

Bragg Liquid Aminos

Mixed fresh herbs, such as parsley, cilantro, or basil

- 1 **lemon, cut into wedges**

Cook quinoa (below) and cook lentils or mung beans separately according to package instructions. Divide quinoa among four bowls. Top with lentils, kale or broccoli, and your choice of tofu, chicken, or salmon, if using. Garnish

How to Cook Quinoa

Use 1 cup quinoa to 2 cups water. Rinse quinoa in a fine-mesh sieve until water runs clear, drain, and transfer to a medium pot. Add water and salt and bring to a boil. Cover, reduce heat to medium low, and simmer until water is absorbed, 15 to 20 minutes. Set aside off the heat 5 minutes; uncover and fluff with a fork.

with avocado. Serve with liquid aminos, herbs, and lemon wedges.

Per serving (does not include optional tofu, chicken, or salmon): 440 calories, 12g total fat, 1.5g saturated fat, 0mg cholesterol, 75mg sodium, 70g total carbohydrate (16g dietary fiber, 3g sugar, 0g added sugars), 21g protein, 2.7mg iron

Pineapple-Ginger Rice Bowl with Edamame
Serves 4

This meal in a bowl is delicious as is or topped with baked tofu, steamed fish, or roasted chicken. If you don't have leftover brown rice on hand, use a package of frozen cooked brown rice as a shortcut.

- ¾ **cup low-sodium vegetable broth**
- 1 **tablespoon finely grated ginger**
- 2 **tablespoons brown rice miso or light yellow miso**

How to Cook Beans

Spread dried beans in a single layer on a large sheet pan; pick through to remove and discard any small stones or debris and then rinse well.

Soak the beans using one of these two methods:

Traditional soaking method: In a large bowl, cover beans by three inches with cold water, cover, and set aside at room temperature 8 hours or overnight.

Quick soaking method: In a large pot, cover beans by three inches with cold water, cover, and bring to a boil. Boil for 1 minute, remove pot from heat, and set aside, covered, 1 hour.

Drain soaked beans and transfer to a large pot. Cover by two inches with cold water, add a couple of bay leaves, and bring to a boil; skim off and discard any foam on the surface. Reduce heat, cover, and simmer, gently stirring occasionally, until beans are tender, 1 to 1½ hours. Drain beans, discard bay leaves, and season with salt. *(Note: Don't add salt before you finish cooking, or it may prevent the beans from softening.)*

4 cups cooked brown rice

2 cups shelled edamame

1½ cups chopped fresh pineapple

¼ cup chopped fresh cilantro

In a large, deep skillet, bring broth and ginger to a simmer over medium-high heat; simmer 2 minutes. Remove skillet from heat and whisk in miso. Return to heat; add rice, edamame, and pineapple; toss gently; and cook until liquid is absorbed and rice is hot throughout, 3 to 5 minutes more. Stir in cilantro and serve.

Per serving: 360 calories (40 from fat), 5g total fat, 0g saturated fat, 0mg cholesterol, 380mg sodium, 66g total carbohydrate (10g dietary fiber, 8g sugar), 14g protein

Austin Taco Bowl

Created by Chad Sarno

Serves 4 to 6

Austin is not only the capital of the Lone Star State and the birthplace of Whole Foods Market, it is also referred to by locals as the taco capital of the States. This bowl is a hearty whole food bowl on its own, or make it more fun and serve with a side of your favorite warmed tortillas.

2 cups fresh or thawed frozen corn off the cob

½ teaspoon ground cumin

1 teaspoon chili powder

1 teaspoon onion granules

3 cups black beans, cooked fresh (see technique, page 288) or 2 (14-ounce) cans no-salt-added black beans (strained and rinsed)

3 cups short-grain brown rice, cooked (see page 286)

½ head romaine lettuce, shredded

1 Red Pepper Pico recipe (see recipe, page 290)

1 Avocado-Jalapeño Crème recipe (see recipe, page 290)

½ cup dry-toasted pumpkin seeds

Hot sauce (optional)

Whole wheat or corn tortillas, warmed (optional)

Preheat oven to 400°F. In a small bowl, add the freshly shucked or thawed corn. Mix with the cumin, chili powder, and onion granules. Spray a baking sheet or line with parchment paper and spread corn evenly. Roast 5 minutes. Remove and allow to cool. Set aside.

To assemble the bowls: Evenly distribute the beans, rice, roasted corn, and lettuce in each bowl. Top each bowl with Red Pepper Pico and Avocado-Jalapeño Crème, and garnish with pumpkin seeds.

Serve with your favorite hot sauce, if you like, and warmed tortillas to assemble your own tacos.

Per serving: 530 calories, 19g total fat, 2.5g saturated fat, 0mg cholesterol, 50mg sodium, 78g total carbohydrate (7g dietary fiber, 8g sugar, 0g added sugars), 20g protein, 3mg iron

Red Pepper Pico

As well as topping the Austin Taco Bowl, this can be served as a salsa.

Makes a bit over 1½ cups

- ½ cup small-diced red bell pepper
- ¾ cup seeded and small-diced Roma tomato
- ¼ cup small-diced red onion
- ½ jalapeño, seeded and finely minced
- 1 tablespoon lime juice
- 1 clove garlic, finely minced
- 3 tablespoons chopped fresh cilantro
- Sea salt to taste

In small mixing bowl, gently toss all ingredients well.

Per serving: 5 calories, 0g total fat, 0g saturated fat, 0mg cholesterol, 0mg sodium, 1g total carbohydrate (0g dietary fiber, 1g sugar, 0g added sugars), 0g protein, 0mg iron

Avocado-Jalapeño Crème

Use as a zesty topping for the Austin Taco Bowl, or serve as a creamy dip.

Makes about 1½ cups

- 2 avocados

2   cloves garlic

2   tablespoons lime juice

1   jalapeño, seeded

¼   cup cilantro, chopped

¼   cup almond or soy milk, unsweetened

Sea salt to taste

In a food processor, blend all ingredients until smooth.

Per serving: 45 calories, 4g total fat, 0g saturated fat, 0mg cholesterol, 0mg sodium, 3g total carbohydrate (1g dietary fiber, 0g sugar, 0g added sugars), 1g protein, 0mg iron

ENTRÉES

Mushroom Stroganoff

Serves 4 to 6

Firm, flavorful mushroom varieties such as cremini, portobello, shiitake, and oyster are ideal for this delicious vegan recipe. It's excellent served over barley.

⅔   cup raw cashews

2   teaspoons red wine vinegar

Pinch fine sea salt

1½   pounds assorted mushrooms

3   shallots, thinly sliced

2½   cups mushroom broth or low-sodium vegetable broth

1   tablespoon Dijon mustard

1   tablespoon paprika

½   teaspoon ground black pepper

3   tablespoons chopped fresh parsley or dill, for garnish

Place cashews in a small bowl and cover by about 1 inch with boiling water. Let soak 30 minutes. Drain, discarding soaking liquid. In a blender, combine cashews, ¼ cup water, vinegar, and salt, and blend until smooth;

add more water, a tablespoon at a time as needed, to make a cashew cream (consistency should be similar to sour cream).

Halve or quarter small mushrooms and thickly slice large ones. Place mushrooms and shallots in a heavy pot and set over medium heat. Cook, stirring frequently, until the mushrooms begin to brown; add broth a few tablespoons at a time to keep mushrooms from sticking to the bottom of the pan. Cook, adding more broth as needed, until mushrooms are browned and softened, 10 to 12 minutes.

Stir in remaining broth, mustard, paprika, and pepper. Bring to a boil, lower heat, and simmer until mushrooms are very tender and sauce is thickened, about 25 minutes. Stir in ½ cup of cashew cream. Sprinkle with parsley and serve with remaining cashew cream on the side.

Per serving: 170 calories, 9g total fat, 1.5g saturated fat, 0mg cholesterol, 380mg sodium, 20g total carbohydrate (2g dietary fiber, 5g sugar, 0g added sugars), 9g protein, 2.7mg iron

Tempeh Curry with Sweet Potatoes and Green Beans

Serves 4

Tempeh absorbs the rich spices and coconut milk in this simple curry. Cook the rice and steam the tempeh while prepping other ingredients and the dish will come together quickly.

- 1 cup long-grain brown rice
- 1 (8-ounce) package tempeh
- 1½ cups low-sodium vegetable broth
- 1 medium yellow onion, chopped
- 2 cloves garlic, finely chopped
- 1 tablespoon freshly grated ginger
- 1 tablespoon curry powder
- 2 teaspoons ground cumin
- 1 (13.5-ounce) can light coconut milk
- 1 large sweet potato, peeled and cut into ½-inch chunks
- ½ pound green beans, trimmed and cut into 1-inch pieces

¼ **cup chopped fresh cilantro**

¼ **teaspoon fine sea salt**

Bring rice and 2 cups water to a boil in a medium saucepan. Reduce heat to low, cover pot, and simmer just until liquid is completely absorbed and rice is tender, about 40 minutes. Meanwhile, arrange steamer basket in a pot. Add just enough water to reach bottom of basket. Bring to a boil. Cut tempeh in half and place in the steamer basket. Reduce heat to medium-low, cover, and steam about 15 minutes or until tender. Remove tempeh and set aside until cool enough to handle. Cut into ½-inch cubes.

Bring ½ cup broth to a simmer in a large deep skillet over medium-high heat. Add onion, garlic, and ginger and cook 5 minutes or until onion is translucent and tender, stirring occasionally. Stir in curry and cumin and cook 1 minute. Add coconut milk, potato, tempeh, and remaining 1 cup broth. Bring to a boil. Reduce heat to medium-low, cover, and cook 10 minutes. Stir in green beans and return to a simmer, uncovered. Cook about 5 minutes longer or until potatoes and green beans are tender. Stir in 3 tablespoons cilantro (keeping 1 tablespoon for garnish) and salt. To serve, spoon curry over rice and garnish with remaining 1 tablespoon cilantro.

Per serving: 530 calories, 12g total fat, 6g saturated fat, 0mg cholesterol, 210mg sodium, 85g total carbohydrate (14g dietary fiber, 10g sugar, 0g added sugars), 26g protein, 6.3mg iron

Indian-Spiced Veggie Burgers

Serves 4

Serve these delicious curry-flavored burgers with cilantro, mango salsa, or sliced avocado. With their rich cashew creaminess, these are quite a calorie-dense meal, so think of them as an occasional treat if you are trying to lose weight.

1 **cup peeled and diced russet potato**

½ **cup small cauliflower florets**

1½ **cups raw unsalted cashews**

½ **cup thawed frozen peas**

continued

⅓ **cup diced green onions**

2 **teaspoons curry powder**

1½ **teaspoons onion granules**

¼ **teaspoon fine sea salt**

¼ **teaspoon ground black pepper**

Cook potato in boiling water until very soft, about 15 minutes. Drain and cool slightly. Cook cauliflower in boiling water until very soft, about 6 minutes. Drain and cool slightly.

Preheat oven to 400°F. Place cashews in a food processor and pulse until finely ground. In a large bowl, combine potato, cauliflower, cashews, and remaining ingredients. Use your hands to break up chunks of potato and cauliflower, and press the ingredients until they hold together. With damp hands, form into patties, about 4 inches in diameter and ¾ inch thick. Place on a parchment paper-lined baking sheet. Bake 15 minutes, then flip burgers and continue to bake until lightly browned on the other side, about 15 minutes longer.

Forming neat veggie burgers: Dampen the inside of a ½-cup measuring cup and pack it with the burger mixture, pressing down firmly. Turn the cup over and shake it gently to release the mixture into the palm of your hand, then press down with your other hand until the patty is about ¾ inch thick.

Freezing and reheating cooked veggie burgers: Cool cooked burgers and wrap individually in plastic wrap and then foil, or place them in

How to Make No-Oil Fries

Preheat oven to 450°F.

Cut potatoes or sweet potatoes into sticks or wedges.

Toss potatoes with a little salt and your favorite herbs or spices (try rosemary, thyme, smoked paprika, cayenne, or cumin).

Spread potatoes in a single layer on a baking sheet lined with parchment paper and bake near the top of the oven until potatoes are browned and cooked through, about 25 minutes.

individual resealable plastic bags and freeze up to 6 months. To reheat, unwrap the burgers, place on a parchment paper-lined baking sheet, and reheat at 300°F until heated through, 20 to 25 minutes.

Per serving (1 burger): 340 calories, 23g total fat, 4g saturated fat, 0mg cholesterol, 180mg sodium, 26g total carbohydrate (4g dietary fiber, 5g sugar, 0g added sugars), 11g protein, 4.5mg iron

Sesame Peanut Noodles

Serves 4

Serve this colorful noodle dish at room temperature or chilled.

- 1 (8-ounce) package 100% whole grain soba noodles
- 2 cups snow peas, strings removed
- 2 tablespoons roasted, unsalted, unsweetened smooth peanut butter or almond butter
- 2 tablespoons rice vinegar
- 1 tablespoon reduced-sodium tamari
- 1 tablespoon sesame tahini
- ⅛ teaspoon crushed red pepper flakes
- 2 cloves garlic, minced or very thinly sliced
- 1½ cups shredded carrots
- 1 red bell pepper, thinly sliced
- 1 bunch green onions, thinly sliced
- 3 tablespoons toasted sesame seeds

Cook soba noodles according to package directions. Add snow peas with 1 minute cooking time remaining. Drain noodles and snow peas thoroughly.

Meanwhile, in a large bowl, whisk together peanut butter, vinegar, tamari, tahini, red pepper flakes, and garlic. Add a splash of warm water if needed to thin the sauce so it will coat the vegetables and noodles. Add noodles, snow peas, carrots, bell pepper, green onions, and sesame seeds. Toss to coat thoroughly. Serve at room temperature or chilled.

Per serving: 400 calories, 12g total fat, 1.5g saturated fat, 0mg cholesterol, 230mg sodium, 59g total carbohydrate (6g dietary fiber, 6g sugar), 11g protein, 7.2mg iron

Jhap Chae Stir-Fry

Created by Derek Sarno

Serves 4

FOR THE COOKING SAUCE

- ¼ cup brown unseasoned rice vinegar
- ¼ cup low-sodium tamari
- 2 dates, pasted (soaked in hot water for one hour and smashed into a paste)
- 1 tablespoon toasted sesame seeds
- 1 tablespoon nori flakes (take a quarter of a nori sheet and crush into fish food-size flakes)
- ½ teaspoon crushed red chili flakes
- ¼ teaspoon smoked paprika
- 1 clove garlic, minced
- ¼ teaspoon coarse sea salt
- ½ teaspoon ground black pepper

- 1 large yellow onion, halved, skin removed, and thinly julienned
- 1 cup shredded Brussels sprouts
- 2 cup julienned shiitake or oyster mushrooms
- Juice of 1 orange (or ¼ cup water)
- 1 pound firm tofu
- Cooking Sauce (above)
- 2 packages (8 ounces) sweet potato noodles or kelp glass noodles or brown rice vermicelli, prepared according to package directions, rinsed and set aside
- 2 carrots, shredded (purple, orange, or yellow)
- ¼ cup fresh cilantro leaves, chopped
- 8 ounces spinach, steamed, cooled, excess water squeezed out, and chopped

Blend all the Cooking Sauce ingredients 2 minutes in a blender.

Heat wok or large sauté pan on medium-high heat, add onions, and dry-sauté (see technique, page 271) 1 minute, then add Brussels sprouts and shiitakes; instead of adding oil, splash ¼ cup water and/or squeeze juice from orange as needed to keep from sticking to the pan and sauté 3 to 5 minutes, stirring frequently until slightly browned and cooked.

Add tofu and Cooking Sauce and cook 3 minutes Bring to quick boil and add noodles and mix together well. Remove from heat.

Serve with shredded carrots and fresh cilantro sprigs, with steamed spinach on the side.

Per serving: 400 calories, 6g total fat, 0.5g saturated fat, 0mg cholesterol, 940mg sodium, 69g total carbohydrate (5g dietary fiber, 14g sugar, 1g added sugars), 19g protein, 7mg iron

Penne Puttanesca with Roasted Red Pepper Sauce

Created by Chad Sarno

Serves 4 to 6

This simple pasta has subtle spiciness and screams flavor with the addition of olives, capers, and fresh herbs. It pairs perfectly with whole grain penne. Also spread this sauce on Pita Pizzas (page 298).

- 8 ounces whole wheat penne
- 1 cup small-diced white onion
- Crushed red chili flakes to taste
- 3 cloves garlic, minced
- ½ cup low-sodium vegetable broth
- 3½ chopped roasted red bell peppers
- ¼ cup pine nuts, dry toasted
- 1 tablespoon balsamic vinegar
- ¼ teaspoon crushed red chili flakes
- 3 tablespoons pitted and chopped kalamata olives
- 3 tablespoons strained capers
- ¼ cup chopped fresh flat leaf parsley
- 3 tablespoons fresh basil chiffonade

Bring a large pot of water to boil for the pasta. Pour in the pasta, stir frequently, and cook until tender, 9 to 11 minutes. Strain.

Place sauté pan on medium to high heat. When pan is heated, add the onion and dry-sauté (see technique, page 271), stirring frequently until onion begins to stick, you begin to see some coloration on the bottom of the pan, and they begin to turn slightly translucent. Add the chili flakes and garlic and cook for 2 minutes, stirring well. Add 2 to 3 tablespoons of vegetable broth to deglaze the pan and remove from heat.

In a blender, add the sautéed onion and garlic, remaining vegetable broth, roasted red peppers, pine nuts, and balsamic vinegar; blend until smooth. Pour pepper puree into a medium saucepan over medium-low heat and slowly bring to a simmer, stirring frequently. Add crushed red chili, olives, capers, parsley, and basil (reserve some fresh herbs for garnish). Stir well and remove from heat. Add in the cooked penne and fold to coat pasta well. Serve hot, garnished with remaining fresh parsley and basil.

Per serving: 280 calories, 10g total fat, 1g saturated fat, 0mg cholesterol, 630mg sodium, 39g total carbohydrate (1g dietary fiber, 7g sugar, 0g added sugars), 10g protein, 4mg iron

Pita Pizza with Herb Pesto and Green Veggies

Created by Chad Sarno

Serves 4

Looking for a quick meal that the kids will love to prepare? Pita pizza night is a way to get creative with sauces and veggies you have on hand for a quick handheld dinner the whole family will enjoy.

   4 to 6 whole wheat pita bread rounds, or Engine 2 Plant-Strong Tortillas (Sprouted Ancient Grain or Brown Rice)

   1 to 1½ cups Oil-Free Herb Pesto (see recipe, page 299)

   1 head of kale, stemmed, lightly steamed, and coarsely chopped
      Small zucchini, sliced on a mandoline in long ribbons

1¼ cups small broccoli florets, lightly steamed

   1 cup Brussels sprout leaves

  ½ cup very thinly sliced onion

  ½ cup sliced olives (optional)

  ½ cup chopped fresh basil

Freshly cracked black pepper

White Balsamic Glaze to finish (optional; see technique, page 282), or Spicy BBQ Tahini Sauce (see recipe, page page 282)

Preheat oven to 400°F. Spray sheet pans lightly with oil or line with parchment paper, and place tortillas or pita bread on pans.

Spread each with about a quarter cup of the herb pesto. Top each pizza with the chopped kale, zucchini ribbons, broccoli, Brussels sprout leaves, shaved onion, olives (if using), and basil.

Place in oven and bake until edges of pitas or tortillas are browned and crisp, about 12 to 15 minutes.

Remove from oven and slice each into 4 to 6 pieces. Finish with cracked black pepper.

Drizzle with White Balsamic Glasze or Spicy BBQ Tahini Sauce before serving.

Recipe note: Looking for more sauces for pizzas? Check out the Penne Puttanesca with Roasted Red Pepper Sauce (see page 297) for a flavor-packed option.

Per serving: 270 calories, 10g total fat, 1.5g saturated fat, 0mg cholesterol, 600mg sodium, 39g total carbohydrate (3g dietary fiber, 5g sugar, 0g added sugars), 13g protein, 4mg iron

Oil-Free Herb Pesto

Makes about 2 cups

2 cups lightly packed chopped basil leaves

¼ cup chopped parsley

¼ cup chopped leeks

2 cloves garlic

½ cup lightly dry-toasted pine nuts

2 tablespoons nutritional yeast

½ avocado, pit and skin removed

½ teaspoon coarse sea salt

In a food processor, add all ingredients. Blend to finely minced, taking off lid and scraping sides as needed. Once the mix is finely minced, add a small amount of water and blend a bit more, leaving some texture so the mixture is not fully smooth. You may need a bit more water to get the thickness you desire for pizzas.

Use on pasta or pizza, or as a spread for sandwiches and wraps.
(Note: If using for pasta, you may need to dilute the sauce a bit more with a splash of vegetable stock, soy milk, or water to thin.)

Per serving (¼ cup): 60 calories, 4.5g total fat, 1g saturated fat, 0mg cholesterol, 150mg sodium, 3g total carbohydrate (0g dietary fiber, 0g sugar, 0g added sugars), 2g protein, 1mg iron

Refried Bean and Avocado Soft Tacos
Serves 4

Perfectly seasoned beans are balanced by the fresh flavors of avocado, lettuce, and tomato for a healthier version of a fast-food favorite. Kick up the heat with your favorite hot sauce!

 1 white onion, finely chopped
 2 cloves garlic, minced
1½ cups low-sodium vegetable broth
 2 (15-ounce) cans no-salt-added pinto beans (about 3 cups), drained and rinsed
1½ teaspoons cumin
 ½ teaspoon fine sea salt
 ¼ teaspoon ground black pepper
 8 corn tortillas
 2 cups shredded romaine lettuce
 3 Roma tomatoes, diced
1½ avocados, thinly sliced

Heat a large skillet over medium heat until hot. Add onion and garlic and cook 3 to 4 minutes or until they begin to stick to the skillet (see dry-sauté technique, page 271). Stir in ½ cup broth and cook 6 to 8 minutes or until onion is translucent and very tender. Reduce heat to medium-low, add beans, and cook 2 to 3 minutes to soften, stirring frequently. Mash beans with a potato masher. Stir in remaining broth, cumin, salt, and pepper. Cook 5 minutes longer or until warmed through, stirring occasionally and adding water or more broth as needed for desired consistency.

In a dry skillet over medium heat, warm each tortilla to soften. Top with a generous scoop of bean mixture. Add lettuce, tomatoes, and avocados. Fold in half and serve with your favorite salsa.

Per serving: 420 calories (110 from fat), 13g total fat, 1.5g saturated fat, 0mg cholesterol, 340mg sodium, 64g total carbohydrate (20g dietary fiber, 5g sugar), 14g protein

Garden Picnic Pasta Salad with Veggies, Herbs, and Orange-MisoTahini Dressing

Created by Derek Sarno

Serves 6 or more

We love this creamy umami bomb of earthy deliciousness for dinner or lunch—and leftovers the next day! It's easy to prepare and can be done the day before so it's ready to go when you want.

  2 small zucchini, thinly sliced into half moons
  2 cups bite-size broccoli florets
  1 cup coarsely diced onion
  3 cups lightly packed bite-size, hand-torn kale (rinsed and cleaned)
  1 pound whole grain or gluten-free fusilli pasta, cooked and rinsed
  1 (14-ounce) can chickpeas, drained and rinsed
  1 cup halved cherry tomatoes
  ¼ cup lightly toasted pine nuts
  ¼ cup lightly packed coarsely chopped parsley
  ¼ cup lightly packed coarsely chopped basil
  1 tablespoon minced garlic
  1½ cups Orange-Miso-Tahini Dressing (see recipe, page 302)

Fill a medium saucepan three-quarters full of water, bring to boil, and add zucchini, broccoli, and onion. Blanch 3 minutes until tender and the colors pop vibrantly. Just before draining, mix in torn kale. Remove from heat, strain, and rinse with cold water until cooled.

In a large bowl, combine freshly cooled, rinsed, and drained pasta, chickpeas, cooked and raw veggies, pine nuts, herbs, garlic, and half the dressing. Mix in additional dressing until creamy and the consistency you like. Save leftover dressing for later use, to refresh, or to serve on the side.

Per serving: 510 calories, 18g total fat, 2g saturated fat, 0mg cholesterol, 350mg sodium, 76g total carbohydrate (5g dietary fiber, 9g sugar, 1g added sugars), 22g protein, 5mg iron

Orange-Miso Tahini Dressing

Makes about 3 cups

- 1 cups tahini
- ½ cup fresh orange juice (from 2 to 3 oranges)
- ½ cup warm water
- ¼ cup white miso

     Juice of 1 lime
- 1 teaspoon minced garlic
- ½ teaspoon crushed red chili flakes
- ½ teaspoon smoked paprika
- ½ teaspoon onion powder
- ¼ cup finely chopped parsley

Add all ingredients to bowl or blender and mix well to incorporate. May be done the night before and can keep in the fridge for a couple weeks.

Per serving (2 tablespoons): 70 calories, 5g total fat, 0.5g saturated fat, 0mg cholesterol, 80mg sodium, 4g total carbohydrate (0g dietary fiber, 1g sugar, 0.5g added sugars), 2g protein, 1mg iron

Garden-Stuffed Potato Cacciatore

Created by Derek Sarno

Serves 4 or more

The delicious cacciatore can be prepared the day before or in a slow cooker the day of.

- 4 large russet potatoes
- 1 onion, diced medium
- 1 medium zucchini, sliced into ½-inch moons

2 bell peppers, 1-inch diced

1 large carrot, cut into ½-inch moons

2 stalks celery, cut into ½-inch pieces

10 ounces white mushrooms, quartered

2 cups halved cherry tomatoes

6 cloves garlic, coarsely chopped

1 teaspoon black pepper

1 bay leaf

½ teaspoon coarse salt

1 tablespoon cumin

1 teaspoon dried oregano or ¼ cup lightly packed fresh leaves

1 (14-ounce) can diced tomatoes (no salt added)

1 cup lightly packed coarsely chopped fresh basil

½ cup roughly chopped flat leaf parsley

2 cups Cashew Sour Cream (see recipe, page 284; add ¼ cup chives, omit jalapeño)

Preheat oven to 375°F. Scrub potatoes and place on a baking pan. Bake 45 minutes or until cooked through (a skewer or knife can easily slide through). Carefully slice each potato in half, leaving the skin intact. Fluff and scoop out some of the flesh to mix with the cacciatore.

In a large skillet or saucepan, water-sauté onion (see technique, page 271), add remaining vegetables (through garlic), and stir to incorporate. Sauté 5 minutes. Add pepper, bay leaf, salt, cumin, and oregano and cook another 5 minutes. Add canned tomatoes, lower the heat to medium low, and cook 20 minutes, stirring occasionally. Stir in fluffed potato flesh.

Take off heat. Stir in fresh basil and parsley.

Cover each potato half with a good portion of cacciatore and a dollop or two of Cashew Sour Cream, and bake 15 minutes more.

Remove from oven. Serve with a green salad.

Per serving: 380 calories, 9g total fat, 1.5g saturated fat, 0mg cholesterol, 270mg sodium, 66g total carbohydrate (8g dietary fiber, 13g sugar, 0g added sugars), 13g protein, 5mg iron

DESSERTS AND SWEETS

Oatmeal-Raisin Cookies
Makes about 2 dozen

These classic gluten-free cookies get natural sweetness from rehydrated raisins. To vary the flavor, add chopped nuts or other dried fruits.

- 1 **cup raisins**
- 1 **cup gluten-free rolled oats**
- 1 **teaspoon baking powder**
- 1 **teaspoon ground cinnamon**
- ¼ **teaspoon ground nutmeg**
- ¼ **teaspoon fine sea salt**
- ½ **cup no-salt-added cashew butter**
- 1 **teaspoon pure vanilla extract**

Preheat oven to 350°F. Line 2 baking sheets with parchment paper. Soak ½ cup of the raisins in warm water at least 10 minutes, leaving the remaining ½ cup dry. Drain and reserve ¼ cup of the soaking liquid. Pulse ¾ cup of the oats in a blender or food processor until finely ground and powdery, setting aside the remaining ¼ cup. (Do not wash the food processor.) In a large bowl, whisk together oat flour, baking powder, cinnamon, nutmeg and salt; set aside. Combine raisins and ¼ cup of the soaking liquid in the food processor. Pulse to chop, then puree until smooth. Add cashew butter and vanilla, then puree until creamy. Add raisin mixture, remaining ½ cup whole raisins, and remaining ¼ cup oats to oat mixture. Stir thoroughly until all the oat flour is absorbed.

Drop heaping teaspoons of dough on the prepared baking sheets, spacing cookies about 1 inch apart. Gently flatten each with the back of a spoon. Bake until cookies are lightly browned on the bottom, 10 to 12 minutes.

Let cookies cool on the baking sheet for 5 minutes, then transfer them to a wire rack and let cool completely. Cookies will keep in an airtight container at room temperature up to 3 days or in the freezer up to 2 weeks.

Per serving (1 cookie): 70 calories, 3g total fat, 0.5g saturated fat, 0mg cholesterol, 45mg sodium, 9g total carbohydrate (1g dietary fiber, 3g sugar, 0g added sugars), 2g protein, 0.6mg iron

Sweet Potato Chocolate Mousse
Serves 4 to 6

This rich vegan mousse gets its silky texture and irresistible sweetness from pureed sweet potatoes. Substitute canned pumpkin or pureed bananas for the sweet potato if you like. Use this mousse as a simple pie filling or layer it with fresh fruit for an easy parfait.

- ¾ cup pitted dates, soaked in warm water 10 minutes to soften
- 2 cups sweet potato purée (fresh or canned)
- 2 tablespoons no-salt-added unsweetened almond butter
- ¾ cup unsweetened almond milk
- ½ cup unsweetened cocoa powder
- ½ teaspoon ground cinnamon
- 1 teaspoon pure vanilla extract
- 3 tablespoons flaxseed meal

Drain soaking liquid from dates, squeeze out any excess water, and place dates in a food processor or high-speed blender. Add sweet potato, almond butter, almond milk, cocoa, cinnamon, vanilla, and flaxseed meal, and puree until well combined and creamy. Refrigerate mousse in an airtight container up to 3 days or freeze up to 5 days.

If using for a pie filling, pour mousse into a baked piecrust. Cover tightly and refrigerate at least 2 hours or overnight before serving.

Per serving (½ cup): 250 calories, 6g total fat, 1.5g saturated fat, 0mg cholesterol, 65mg sodium, 49g total carbohydrate (10g dietary fiber, 24g sugar, 0g added sugars), 6g protein, 1.8mg iron

Raspberry Nice Cream

Serves 4

With a little blender and freezer magic, raspberries, bananas, and rich cashews become a sweet and flavorful "ice cream."

- 6 ounces raspberries, fresh or frozen and thawed
- ½ cup raw whole cashews, soaked in warm water at room temperature at least 2 hours, drained
- 2 bananas, peeled, thickly sliced, and frozen

Puree raspberries and cashews in a blender or food processor until smooth, adding up to ¼ cup water if needed to puree. Add bananas and puree again, scraping down the sides often, until very smooth.

Transfer to a tightly sealed freezer-safe container and freeze until just solid, about 4 hours. (If you make far in advance, soften at room temperature 15 minutes before scooping.)

Per serving (about ½ cup): 170 calories, 8g total fat, 1.5g saturated fat, 0mg cholesterol, 0mg sodium, 26g total carbohydrate (2g dietary fiber, 11g sugar, 0g added sugars), 4g protein, 1.4mg iron

WHOLE FOODIE HEROES: HONORABLE MENTIONS

Throughout these pages we've honored a few of our Whole Foodie Heroes. However, there was not enough space for all the people who have influenced us, inspired us, and helped to grow the whole foods, plant-based eating movement. Here are some more of those people:

- **Chef AJ**—Plant-based chef, host of *Healthy Living with Chef AJ*
- **Nelson Campbell**—Creator and director of the film *PlantPure Nation*
- **Linda Carney, MD**—Plant-based physician, educator
- **Paul Chatlin**—Founder, Plant-Based Nutrition Support Group
- **Karen Dawn**—Animal rights activist, author of *Thanking the Monkey: Rethinking the Way We Treat Animals*
- **Ann Esselstyn**—Plant-based educator and chef
- **Gary Fraser**—Professor of epidemiology, principal researcher in the Adventist Heath Studies
- **Kathy Freston**—Health and wellness expert, author of *The Book of Veganish*
- **Bruce Friedrich**—Animal rights activist, founder of the Good Food Institute
- **Julieanna Hever**—Plant-based dietitian, author of *The Complete Idiot's Guide to Plant-Based Nutrition*
- **Scott Jurek**—Ultra-athlete, author of *Eat and Run: My Unlikely Journey to Ultramarathon Greatness*
- **Joel Kahn, MD**—Plant-based cardiologist, author of *The Whole Heart Solution*
- **Terry Mason, MD**—Plant-based physician, public health official
- **Craig McDougall, MD**—Plant-based physician, Zoom+Prime

- **Milton Mills, MD**—Plant-based speaker and educator
- **Baxter Montgomery, MD**—Plant-based cardiologist, founder of Montgomery Heart & Wellness
- **Lani Muelrath**—Plant-based educator, author of *The Plant-Based Journey* and *The Mindful Vegan (Fall 2017)*
- **Marion Nestle**—Professor of nutrition, author of *Food Politics*
- **Ocean Robbins**—cofounder and CEO of the Food Revolution Network
- **Rich Roll**—Plant-based athlete, author, host of The Rich Roll Podcast
- **Will Tuttle**—Musician, educator, author of *The World Peace Diet*
- **Alice Waters**—Owner of Chez Panisse, pioneer of California cuisine
- **Brian Wendel**—Creator of the Forks over Knives franchise
- **Akua Woolbright, PhD**—Senior healthy eating and wellness educator, Whole Cities Foundation

ACKNOWLEDGMENTS

We want to especially thank Ellen Daly and Carter Phipps, who did most of the heavy lifting on this book for several months. Without their help, dedication, and superb writing skills, we doubt this book would have been even half as good as it turned out to be.

Special thanks to Dr. Dean Ornish for writing the Foreword and for the incredible work he has done, proving to the world that heart disease is both a preventable and reversible disease through lifestyle change, including eating a low-fat, whole foods, plant-based diet.

We owe so much to all of our Whole Foodie Heroes for all they have taught us. If we have seen further than many people do, it is only because we have been standing on the shoulders of these giants. Special thanks to those who shared their time to give us personal interviews and advice: T. Colin Campbell, Michael Pollan, John McDougall, Dean Ornish, Joel Fuhrman, Michael Greger, Rip Esselstyn, Neal Barnard, Dan Buettner, Kathy Freston, Joel Kahn, Garth Davis, Pam Popper, Lani Muelrath, Akua Woolbright, Paul Chatlin, and Jeff Novick.

We want to thank Chad Sarno, Derek Sarno, Tien Ho, Molly Siegler, and Jess Kolko for the many wonderful recipes included in this book and Derek again for his excellent food photography.

Our gratitude also goes to the Whole Foods Market team members and PBNSG members who shared their inspirational stories with us: Rebeca Atkins, Russell Cartwright, Shannon Farrell, David Henderson, Marty Jenkins, Milan Ross, Debbie Schafer, Frank Schuck, and Adam Sud.

We want to thank our agent Richard Pine, as well as Eliza Rothstein, at Inkwell, for their dedicated work shepherding our book along. Sarah Pelz, our editor at Grand Central, was both an excellent editor who turned around our work extremely fast, and also proved to be open and flexible to our many requests.

Of course, we want to thank our colleagues at Whole Foods Market who have supported our work in numerous ways, including Walter Robb, Glenda Flanagan, A.C. Gallo, Jim Sud, David Lannon, Ken Meyer, Jason Beuchel, Betsy Foster, Evening Galvin, Falesha Thrash, Bobby Covington, Brook Buchanan, Robin Rehfield Kelly, Martin Tracey, and Sonya Gafsi Oblisk.

Finally we want to thank our families who provide the support and love that makes our work possible.

John: I especially want to thank my wife, Deborah, who is the great love of my life and who committed to share with me this grand adventure called life.

Matt and Alona: We want to thank our daughters, Kylee and Jordan, for ever inspiring us to do better and be better.

ENDNOTES

Introduction by John Mackey

1   2015, "About the National Action Plan," National Fruit and Vegetable Alliance, accessed September 2016, http://www.nfva.org/national_action_plan.html.
2   Economic Research Service, United States Department of Agriculture: Loss Adjusted Food Availability. https://www.ers.usda.gov/data products/food availability per capita data system/summary findings/, accessed Nov. 2016.
3   2014, "Obesity and Overweight," Centers for Disease Control and Prevention, accessed September 2016, http://www.cdc.gov/nchs/fastats/obesity overweight.htm.

PART I. THE WHOLE TRUTH: WHAT WE KNOW ABOUT DIET AND HEALTH

Chapter 1. Are You a Whole Foodie? Defining the Optimum Diet

1   2014, "Obesity and Overweight," Centers for Disease Control and Prevention, accessed September 2016, http://www.cdc.gov/nchs/fastats/obesity overweight.htm.
2   Cynthia L. Ogden, PhD, and Margaret D. Carroll, MSPH, 2010, "Prevalence of Overweight, Obesity, and Extreme Obesity Among Adults: United States, Trends 1960–1962 through 2007–2008," Centers for Disease Control and Prevention, http://www.cdc.gov/nchs/data/hestat/obesity_adult_07_08/obesity_adult_07_08.pdf.
3   2014, "Childhood Obesity Facts," Centers for Disease Control and Prevention, accessed September 2016, http://www.cdc.gov/obesity/data/childhood.html.
4   *National Diabetes Statistics Report*, Centers for Disease Control and Prevention, http://www.cdc.gov/diabetes/pubs/statsreport14/national diabetes report web.pdf.
5   OECD, *Health at a Glance 2015: OECD Indicators* (Paris: OECD Publishing, 2015).
6   Sharada Keats and Steve Wiggins, *Future Diets: Implications for Agriculture and Food Prices*, ODI, accessed September 2016, https://www.odi.org/future diets.
7   John Skell, "Lean Times for the Diet Industry," *Fortune*, May 22, 2015, http://fortune.com/2015/05/22/lean times for the diet industry/.
8   Marketdata Enterprises Inc., Number of American Dieters Soars to 108 Million; Market to Grow 4.5% to $65 Billion in 2012 (press release).
9   Margaret Sanger Katz, "America Starts to Push Away from the Plate," *The New York Times*, July 26, 2015, A1.
10   *2012 Food & Health Survey*, International Food Information Council Foundation, http://www.foodinsight.org/Content/3848/FINAL%202012%20Food%20and%20Health%20Exec%20Summary.pdf.
11   Patrick J. Skerrett and Walter C. Willett, "Essentials of Healthy Eating: A Guide," *Journal of Midwifery & Women's Health* 55 (6) (2010): 492–501. http://www.ncbi.nlm.nih.gov/pmc/articles/PMC3471136/pdf/nihms242610.pdf.
12   David Katz and Stephanie Meller, "Can We Say What Diet Is Best for Health?" *Annual Review of Public Health* 35 (2014): 83–103.
13   "Oldways Common Ground Consensus Statement on Healthy Eating," Oldways, accessed September 2016, http://oldwayspt.org/common ground consensus.
14   2015, "About the National Action Plan," National Fruit and Vegetable Alliance, accessed September 2016, downloaded from: http://www.nfva.org/national_action_plan.html.
15   David L. Katz, MD, MPH, "Diets, Doubts, and Doughnuts: Are We TRULY Clueless?" *The Huffington Post*, August 13, 2016, http://www.huffingtonpost.com/entry/diets doubts and doughnuts are we truly clueless_us_57af2fe9e4b0ae60ff029f0d.
16   Ibid.
17   Michael Greger, *How Not to Die: Discover the Foods Scientifically Proven to Prevent and Reverse Disease* (New York: Macmillan, 2015), 263.
18   Michael Pollan, *Food Rules: An Eater's Manual* (New York: Penguin, 2009), xv.

19   Ibid., 41.
20   Megan Kimble, *Unprocessed: My City Dwelling Year of Reclaiming Real Food* (New York: William Morrow, 2015), 2.
21   Greger, *How Not to Die*, 264.
22   T. Colin Campbell, *Whole: Rethinking the Science of Nutrition*, (Dallas, TX: BenBella Books, 2013), xiii.
23   G. Bjelakovic, D. Nikolova, R. G. Simonetti, and C. Gluud, "Antioxidant Supplements for Prevention of Gastrointestinal Cancers: A Systematic Review and Meta Analysis," *Lancet*, 364 (9441) (2004): 1219–1228. http://www.thelancet.com/journals/lancet/article/PIIS0140 6736(04)17138 9/abstract.
24   Michael Pollan, "Unhappy Meals," *New York Times Magazine*, January 28, 2007. http://www.nytimes.com/2007/01/28/magazine/28nutritionism.t.html.

Chapter 2. Calorie Rich, Nutrient Poor: Obesity, Chronic Disease, and the Modern Dietary Dilemma

1   Danielle Dellorto, "Global Report: Obesity Bigger Health Crisis Than Hunger," CNN, December 10, 2014, http://www.cnn.com/2012/12/13/health/global burden report/, accessed November 2016
2   2014, "Obesity and Overweight," Centers for Disease Control and Prevention, accessed September 2016, http://www.cdc.gov/nchs/fastats/obesity overweight.htm.
3   2014, "Childhood Obesity Facts," Centers for Disease Control and Prevention, accessed September 2016, http://www.cdc.gov/obesity/data/childhood.html.
4   National Diabetes Statistics Report, Centers for Disease Control and Prevention, http://www.cdc.gov/diabetes/pubs/statsreport14/national diabetes report web.pdf.
5   United States Department of Agriculture, Economic Research Service Food Availability (Per Capita) Data System, Loss Adjusted Food Availability, https://www.ers.usda.gov/data products/food availability per capita data system/summary findings/, accessed September 2016.
6   USA Department of Agriculture Economic Research Service, https://www.ers.usda.gov/data products/food availability per capita data system/summary findings/, accessed November 2016.
7   Economic Research Service, United States Department of Agriculture: Loss Adjusted Food Availability. https://www.ers.usda.gov/data products/food availability per capita data system/summary findings/, accessed November 2016.
8   Brady Dennis, "Nearly 60 percent of Americans—the highest ever—are taking prescription drugs," the *Washington Post*, November 3, 2015, https://www.washingtonpost.com/news/to your health/wp/2015/11/03/more americans than ever are taking prescription drugs/.
9   Walter C. Willett, MD, *Eat, Drink, and Be Healthy: The Harvard Medical School Guide to Healthy Eating* (New York: Free Press, 2001), 35.
10   2016, "Obesity and Overweight," World Health Organization, accessed September 2016, http://www.who.int/mediacentre/factsheets/fs311/en/.
11   J. H. Ledikwe et al., "Dietary energy density is associated with energy intake and weight status in US adults," *American Journal of Clinical Nutrition* 83 (6) (2006): 1362–1368.
12   Joel Fuhrman, MD, *The End of Dieting: How to Live for Life* (San Francisco: HarperOne, 2015), 30.
13   Joel Fuhrman, *Super Immunity: The Essential Nutrition Guide for Boosting Your Body's Defenses to Live Longer, Stronger, and Disease Free* (San Francisco: HarperOne, 2011), 12.
14   Joel Fuhrman, MD, in conversation with the authors, July 2016.
15   R. J. Joseph et al., "The Neurocognitive Connection between Physical Activity and Eating Behavior," *Obesity Reviews* 12 (10) (2011): 800–812, doi:10.1111/j.1467 789X.2011.00893.x.
16   Veleba J, Matoulek M, Hill M, Pelikanova T, Kahleova H, "A vegetarian vs. conventional hypocaloric diet: the effect on physical fitness in response to aerobic exercise in patients with type 2 diabetes. A parallel randomized study," *Nutrients*. 2016;8:pii:E671.

Chapter 3. Connecting Diet and Disease: Nutritional Science Looks at the Big Picture

1   A. Wolk, "Potential Health Hazards of Eating Red Meat," *Journal of Internal Medicine* (2016): doi: 10.1111/joim.12543. http://onlinelibrary.wiley.com/doi/10.1111/joim.12543/full.
2   W. B. Grant, "A Multicountry Ecological Study of Cancer Incidence Rates in 2008 with Respect to Various Risk Modifying Factors," *Nutrients* 6 (1) (2013): 163–189.
3   Susanna C. Larsson and Nicola Orsini, "Red Meat and Processed Meat Consumption and All Cause Mortality: A Meta Analysis," *American Journal of Epidemiology* 179 (3) (2014): 282–289, doi:10.1093/aje/kwt261; Levine, Morgan E. et al., "Low Protein Intake Is Associated with a Major Reduction in IGF 1, Cancer, and Overall Mortality in the 65 and Younger but Not Older Population," *Cell Metabolism* 19 (3), (2014) 407–417; M. Song et al., "Association of Animal and Plant Protein Intake with All Cause and Cause Specific Mortality," *JAMA Internal Medicine* 176 (10) (2016): 1453–1463, doi:10.1001/jamainternmed.2016.4182.
4   *Red Meat, Processed Red Meats and the Prevention of Colorectal Cancer*, Publication of the Superior Health Council No. 8858, December 4, 2013.

5   2015, "Q&A on the Carcinogenicity of the Consumption of Red Meat and Processed Meat," World Health Organization, accessed September 2016, http://www.who.int/features/qa/cancer red meat/en/.

6   World Cancer Research Fund International/American Institute for Cancer Research. "Food, Nutrition, Physical Activity, and the Prevention of Cancer: a Global Perspective." Washington DC: AICR, 2007, 11. http://www.aicr.org/assets/docs/pdf/reports/Second_Expert_Report.pdf, accessed September 2016.

7   Jane E. Brody, "Huge Study of Diet Indicts Fat and Meat," *The New York Times*, May 8, 1990, http://www.nytimes.com/1990/05/08/science/huge study of diet indicts fat and meat.html.

8   T. Colin Campbell, PhD, and Thomas M. Campbell II, MD, *The China Study: The Most Comprehensive Study of Nutrition Ever Conducted and the Startling Implications for Diet, Weight Loss, and Long Term Health* (Dallas, TX: BenBella Books, 2005), 7.

9   Tara Parker Pope, "Nutrition Advice from the China Study," *Well* (blog), *The New York Times*, January 7, 2011, http://well.blogs.nytimes.com/2011/01/07/nutrition advice from the china study/.

10   Ibid.

11   Ibid.

12   Campbell and Campbell, *China Study*, 7.

13   Dan Buettner, *The Blue Zones Solution: Eating and Living Like the World's Healthiest People,* (Washington DC: National Geographic, 2015), 66.

14   Emily Esfahani Smith, "The Lovely Hill Where People Live Longer and Happier," *Atlantic*, February 4, 2013, http://www.theatlantic.com/health/archive/2013/02/the lovely hill where people live longer and happier/272798/.

15   Buettner, *Blue Zones Solution*, 65.

16   *Adventist Health Studies: An Overview*, Loma Linda University, https://publichealth.llu.edu/sites/publichealth.llu.edu/files/docs/sph ahs overview.pdf.

17   Buettner, *Blue Zones Solution*, 65.

18   M. J. Orlich et al., "Vegetarian Dietary Patterns and Mortality in Adventist Health Study 2," *JAMA Internal Medicine* 173 (13) (2013): 1230–1238, doi:10.1001/jamainternmed.2013.6473.

19   Serena Tonstad, MD, PhD, DRPH, Ru Yan, MSC, Terry Butler, DRPH, and Gary E. Fraser, MD, PhD, "Type of Vegetarian Diet, Body Weight, and Prevalence of Type 2 Diabetes," *Diabetes Care* 32 (5) (2009): 791–796.

20   David Blumenthal, "Academic Industrial Relationships in the Life Sciences," *New England Journal of Medicine* 25 (349) (2003): 2452–2459; and Agence France Presse (AFP), June 2006.

21   P. J. Tuso et al., "Nutritional Update for Physicians: Plant Based Diets," *Permanente Journal* 17 (2) (2013): 61–66, doi: 10.7812/TPP/12 085; Kate Marsh, Carol Zeuschner, and Angela Saunders, "Health Implications of a Vegetarian Diet: A Review" *American Journal of Lifestyle Medicine* 6 (250) (2012, originally published online November 4, 2011): 250 267, doi: 10.1177/1559827611425762.

22   K.T. Khaw et al., "Combined Impact of Health Behaviours and Mortality in Men and Women: The EPIC Norfolk Prospective Population Study," *PLOS Medicine* 5 (1) (2008): e12. doi: 10.1371/journal.pmed.0050012.

23   Garth Davis, MD, in conversation with the authors, February 2016.

Chapter 4. Reverse-Engineering Longevity: Food and Culture in the Blue Zones

1   E. B. Rubin, A. E. Buehler, S. D. Halpern, "States Worse than Death among Hospitalized Patients with Serious Illnesses," *JAMA Internal Medicine*, published online August 01, 2016, doi:10.1001/jamainternmed.2016.4362.

2   Dan Buettner, in conversation with the authors, July 2016.

3   Ibid.

4   A. M. Herskind et al., "The Heritability of Human Longevity: A Population Based Study of 2872 Danish Twin Pairs Born 1870–1900, *Human Genetics* 97 (3) (1996): 319–323.

5   Buettner, *Blue Zones Solution*, 37.

6   Ibid., 73.

7   Dan Buettner, in conversation with the authors, July 2016.

8   Ibid.

9   Luis Rosero Bixby, William H. Dow, and David H. Rehkopf, "The Nicoya Region of Costa Rica: A High Longevity Island for Elderly Males," *Vienna Yearbook of Population Research/Vienna Institute of Demography, Austrian Academy of Sciences* 11 (2013): 109–136.

10   Dan Buettner, in conversation with the authors, July 2016.

11   Buettner, *Blue Zones Solution*, 179.

12   Dan Buettner, in conversation with the authors, July 2016.

13   Ibid.

14   Ibid.

15   Ibid.

16   J. Connor, "Alcohol Consumption as a Cause of Cancer," *Addiction* (2016), doi: 10.1111/add.13477. http://onlinelibrary.wiley.com/doi/10.1111/add.13477/abstract.

Chapter 5. Let Food Be Thy Medicine: Using Diet to Prevent and Reverse Heart Disease

1   "Heart Disease, Stroke and Research Statistics At a Glance," American Heart Association and American Stroke Association, https://www.heart.org/idc/groups/ahamah public/@wcm/@sop/@smd/documents/downloadable/ucm_480086.pdf.

2   Paul Chatlin, in conversation with the authors, May 2016.

3   W. F. Enos, Jr., R. H. Holmes, and J. Beyer, "Coronary Disease among United States Soldiers Killed in Action in Korea: Preliminary Report," *Journal of the American Medical Association* 152 (12) (1953): 1090–1093, doi:10.1001/jama.1953.03690120006002; J. P. Strong, "Landmark Perspective: Coronary Atherosclerosis in Soldiers. A Clue to the Natural History of Atherosclerosis in the Young," *Journal of the American Medical Association* 256 (20) (1986): 2863–2866; W. F. Enos Jr., J. C. Beyer, and R. H. Holmes, "Pathogenesis of Coronary Disease in American Soldiers Killed in Korea," *Journal of the American Medical Association* 158 (11) (1955): 912–914.

4   J. P. Strong and H. C. McGill, "The Pediatric Aspects of Atherosclerosis," *International Journal for Research and Investigation on Atherosclerosis and Related Diseases* 9 (3) (1969): 251–265; C. Napoli et al., "Fatty Streak Formation Occurs in Human Fetal Aortas and Is Greatly Enhanced by Maternal Hypercholesterolemia. Intimal Accumulation of Low Density Lipoprotein and Its Oxidation Precede Monocyte Recruitment into Early Atherosclerotic Lesions," *Journal of Clinical Investigation* 100 (11) (1997): 2680–2690; G. S. Berenson, S. R. Srinivasan, T. A. Nicklas, "Atherosclerosis: A Nutritional Disease of Childhood," *American Journal of Cardiology* 82 (10B) (1998): 22T–29T.

5   D. Ornish, "A Conversation with the Editor," *American Journal of Cardiology*. 90 (3) (2002) 271 298.

6   D.M. Ornish, A.M. Gotto, R.R. Miller, et al., "Effects Of a Vegetarian Diet and Selected Yoga Techniques in the Treatment of Coronary Heart Disease," *Clinical Research*. 1979; 27:720A.

7   Caldwell Esselstyn, MD, *Prevent and Reverse Heart Disease: The Revolutionary, Scientifically Proven, Nutrition Based Cure* (New York: Avery, 2008), 17.

8   D. Ornish et al., "Can Lifestyle Changes Reverse Coronary Heart Disease?" *Lancet* 336 (8708) (1990): 129–133.

9   D. Ornish, L. W. Scherwitz, J. H. Billings et al., "Intensive Lifestyle Changes for Reversal of Coronary Heart Disease," *Journal of the American Medical Association* 280 (23) (1998): 2001–2007, doi:10.1001/jama.280.23.2001; K.L. Gould, D. Ornish, L. Scherwitz, et al. "Changes In Myocardial Perfusion Abnormalities By Positron Emission Tomography After Long Term, Intense Risk Factor Modification, *JAMA* 274 (11) (1995) 894 901.

10   Esselstyn, *Prevent and Reverse Heart Disease,* 54 55.

11   C. B. Esselstyn Jr. et al., "A Way to Reverse CAD?" *Journal of Family Practice* 63 (7) (2014): 356 364.

12   Dean Ornish, MD, in conversation with the authors, June 2016.

13   Kim A. Williams, MD, 2014, "Vegan Diet, Healthy Heart?" *MedPage Today* and the American Heart Association, http://www.medpagetoday.com/Blogs/CardioBuzz/46860.

14   Dean Ornish, in conversation with the authors, June 2016.

15   Michael Greger, in conversation with the authors, February 2016.

16   Kai Kupferschmidt, "Scientists Fix Errors in Controversial Paper about Saturated Fats," *Science*, March 24, 2014, http://www.sciencemag.org/news/2014/03/scientists fix errors controversial paper about saturated fats.

17   David Katz, "Is All Saturated Fat the Same?" *Huffington Post*, August 14, 2011, http://www.huffingtonpost.com/david katz md/saturated fat_b_875401.html.

18   David Katz, "My Milk Manifesto," *Huffington Post*, March 2, 2015, http://www.huffingtonpost.com/david katz md/my milk manifesto_b_6786048.html.

19   Paul Chatlin, in conversation with the authors, May 2016.

20   Joel Kahn, MD, in conversation with the authors, May 2016.

21   Ibid.

22   Paul Chatlin, in conversation with the authors, May 2016.

23   Ibid.

24   Akua Woolbright, in conversation with the authors, May 2016.

Chapter 6. The Epidemic of Our Time: Demystifying Diabetes

1   *National Diabetes Statistics Report*, Centers for Disease Control and Prevention, http://www.cdc.gov/diabetes/pubs/statsreport14/national diabetes report web.pdf.

2   A. G. Tabák, C. Herder, W. Rathmann, E.J. Brunner, & M. Kivimäki, "Prediabetes: A High Risk State for Developing Diabetes," *Lancet*, 379(9833) (2012): 2279–2290. http://doi.org/10.1016/S0140 6736(12)60283 9.

3   Neal Barnard, MD, *Dr. Neal Barnard's Program for Reversing Diabetes: The Scientifically Proven System for Reversing Diabetes without Drugs* (New York: Rodale, 2006), 16.

4   B. Hemmingsen et al., "Intensive Glycaemic Control for Patients with Type 2 Diabetes: Systematic

Review with Meta Analysis and Trial Sequential Analysis of Randomised Clinical Trials," *BMJ* 343 (d6898) (2011). doi: 10.1136/bmj.d6898.

5   H. C. Gerstein et al., "Effects of Intensive Glucose Lowering in Type 2 Diabetes," *New England Journal of Medicine* 358 (24) (2008): 2545–2559, doi: 10.1056/NEJMoa0802743.

6   R. Rodríguez Gutiérrez and V. M. Montori, "Glycemic Control for Patients with Type 2 Diabetes Mellitus: Our Evolving Faith in the Face of Evidence," *Circulation: Cardiovascular Quality and Outcomes* 9 (5) (2016): 504–512, doi:10.1161/CIRCOUTCOMES.116.002901.

7   Neal Barnard, MD, in conversation with the authors, May 2016.

8   Ibid.

9   M. Roden et al., "Mechanism of Free Fatty Acid Induced Insulin Resistance in Humans." *Journal of Clinical Investigation* 97 (12) (1996): 2859–2865; M. Krssak et al., "Intramyocellular Lipid Concentrations Are Correlated with Insulin Sensitivity in Humans: A 1H NMR Spectroscopy Study," *Diabetologia* 42 (1) (1999): 113–116; A. V. Greco et al., "Insulin Resistance in Morbid Obesity: Reversal with Intramyocellular Fat Depletion," *Diabetes* 51 (1) (2002): 144–151; L. M. Sparks et al., "A High Fat Diet Coordinately Downregulates Genes Required for Mitochondrial Oxidative Phosphorylation in Skeletal Muscle," *Diabetes* 54 (7) (2005): 1926–1933.

10   A. T. Santomauro et al., "Overnight Lowering of Free Fatty Acids with Acipimox Improves Insulin Resistance and Glucose Tolerance in Obese Diabetic and Nondiabetic Subjects," *Diabetes* 48 (9) (1999) 1836–1841, doi: 10.2337/diabetes.48.9.1836; A. V. Greco et al. "Insulin Resistance in Morbid Obesity: Reversal with Intramyocellular Fat Depletion," *Diabetes* 51 (1) (2002): 144–151; M. Roden et al., "Mechanism of Free Fatty Acid–Induced Insulin Resistance in Humans," *Journal of Clinical Investigation* 97 (12) (1996): 2859–2865.

11   Neal Barnard et al., "A Low Fat Vegan Diet and a Conventional Diabetes Diet in the Treatment of Type 2 Diabetes: A Randomized, Controlled, 74 Wk Clinical Trial," *American Journal of Clinical Nutrition* 89 (5) (2009): 1588S–1596S.

12   D. A. Snowdon and R. L. Phillips, "Does a Vegetarian Diet Reduce the Occurrence of Diabetes?" *American Journal of Public Health* 75 (5) (1985): 507–512.

13   S. Tonstad et al., "Vegetarian Diets and Incidence of Diabetes in the Adventist Health Study 2." *Nutrition, Metabolism, and Cardiovascular Diseases : NMCD* 23 (4) (2013): 292–299.

14   U. Smith, "Carbohydrates, Fat, and Insulin Action," *American Journal of Clinical Nutrition* 59 (3 Suppl) (1994): 686S–689S; T. G. Kiehm, J. W. Anderson, and K. Ward, "Beneficial Effects of a High Carbohydrate, High Fiber Diet on Hyperglycemic Diabetic Men," *American Journal of Clinical Nutrition* 29 (8) (1976): 895–899; J. D. Brunzell et al., "Improved Glucose Tolerance with High Carbohydrate Feeding in Mild Diabetes," *New England Journal of Medicine* 284 (10) (1971): 521–524; R. W. Simpson et al., "Improved Glucose Control in Maturity Onset Diabetes Treated with High Carbohydrate Modified Fat Diet," *BMJ* (1979): 1753–1756; J. W. Anderson and K. Ward, "High Carbohydrate, High Fiber Diets for Insulin Treated Men with Diabetes Mellitus," *American Journal of Clinical Nutrition* 32 (11) (1979): 2312–2321.

15   Q. Sun et al., "White Rice, Brown Rice, and Risk of Type 2 Diabetes in US Men and Women," *Archives of Internal Medicine* 170 (11) (2010): 961–969, doi: 10.1001/archinternmed.2010.109.

16   Robert E. Post, MD, MS, Arch G. Mainous III, PhD, Dana E. King, MD, MS, and Kit N. Simpson, DrPH et al., "Dietary Fiber for the Treatment of Type 2 Diabetes Mellitus: A Meta Analysis," *J Am Board Fam MedJournal of the American Board of Family Medicine.* 2012;25 (1) (2012): 16 –23.

17   S. H. Holt, J. C. Miller, and P. Petocz, "An Insulin Index of Foods: The Insulin Demand Generated by 1000 kJ Portions of Common Foods," *American Journal of Clinical Nutrition* 66 (5) (1997): 1264–1276; D. Rabinowitz, T. J. Merimee, R. Maffezzoli, and J. A. Burgess, "Patterns of Hormonal Release after Glucose, Protein, and Glucose Plus Protein," *Lancet* 2 (7461) (1966): 454–456.

18   Y. Yokoyama, N. D. Barnard, S. M. Levin, and M. Watanabe, "Vegetarian Diets and Glycemic Control in Diabetes: A Systematic Review and Meta Analysis," *Cardiovascular Diagnosis and Therapy* 4 (5) (2014): 373–382, doi: 10.3978/ j.issn.2223 3652.2014.10.04.

19   Neal D. Barnard et al., "A Low Fat Vegan Diet Improves Glycemic Control and Cardiovascular Risk Factors in a Randomized Clinical Trial in Individuals With Type 2 Diabetes," *Diabetes Care* 29 (8) (2006): 1777–1783, doi: 10.2337/dc06 0606.

20   Riitta Törrönen et al., "Postprandial Glucose, Insulin, and Free Fatty Acid Responses to Sucrose Consumed with Blackcurrants and Lingonberries in Healthy Women," *American Journal of Clinical Nutrition* 96 (3) (2012): 527–533, doi:10.3945/ajcn.112.042184; R. Törrönen et al., "Berries Reduce Postprandial Insulin Responses to Wheat and Rye Breads in Healthy Women," *Journal of Nutrition* 143 (4) (2013): 430–436, doi: 10.3945/jn.112.169771.

21   Allan S. Christensen, Lone Viggers, Kjeld Hasselström, and Søren Gregersen, "Effect of Fruit Restriction on Glycemic Control in Patients with Type 2 Diabetes—A Randomized Trial," *Nutrition Journal* 12 (29) (2013).

22   Amanda Fiegl, "Global Checkup: Most People Living Longer, but Sicker," *National Geographic News*, December 14, 2012, http://news.nationalgeographic.com/news/2012/12/121213 global health disease life expectancy nutrition.

23   Neal Barnard, MD, in conversation with the authors, May 2016.

24   Garth Davis, MD and Howard Jacobson, *Proteinaholic: How Our Obsession with Meat Is Killing Us and What We Can Do about It* (New York: HarperCollins, 2015), 63.

25   Carl B. Frederick, Kaisa Snellman, and Robert D. Putnam, "Increasing Socioeconomic Disparities in Adolescent Obesity," *Proceedings of the National Academy of Sciences* 111 (4) (2014): 1338–1342, doi:10.1073/pnas.1321355110.

Chapter 7. The Great Grain Robbery: Rethinking the Low-Carb Trend

1   *Health, United States, 2015: With Special Feature on Racial and Ethnic Health Disparities*, National Center for Health Statistics, http://www.cdc.gov/nchs/data/hus/hus15.pdf#056.

2   *Dietary Reference Intakes for Energy, Carbohydrate, Fiber, Fat, Fatty Acids, Cholesterol, Protein, and Amino Acids, National Academies of Sciences*, https://www.nationalacademies.org/hmd/Reports/2002/Dietary Reference Intakes for Energy Carbohydrate Fiber Fat Fatty Acids Cholesterol Protein and Amino Acids.aspx.

3   Teresa T. Fung, ScD, et al., "Low Carbohydrate Diets and All Cause and Cause Specific Mortality: Two Cohort Studies," *Annals of Internal Medicine* 153 (5) (2010): 289 298; A. Trichopoulou et al., "Low Carbohydrate–High Protein Diet and Long Term Survival in a General Population Cohort," *European Journal of Clinical Nutrition* 61 (5) (2007): 575–581; Hiroshi Noto, Atsushi Goto, Tetsuro Tsujimoto, Mitsuhiko Noda, "Low Carbohydrate Diets and All Cause Mortality: A Systematic Review and Meta Analysis of Observational Studies," *PLOS ONE* 8 (1) e55030, 2013.

4   John McDougall, MD, "For the Love of Grains," *McDougall Newsletter*, January 2008, https://www.drmcdougall.com/misc/2008nl/jan/grains.htm.

5   John A. McDougall and Mary McDougall, *The Starch Solution: Eat the Foods You Love, Regain Your Health, and Lose the Weight for Good!* (New York: Rodale Books, 2013), 8.

6   John McDougall, in conversation with the authors, September 2016.

7   Philip Klemmer, Clarence E. Grim, and Friedrich C. Luft "Who and What Drove Walter Kempner? The Rice Diet Revisited," *Hypertension* 64 (4) (2014): 684–688. doi: 10.1161/HYPERTENSIONAHA.114.03946.

8   John McDougall et al., "Effects of 7 Days on an Ad Libitum Low Fat Vegan Diet: The McDougall Program Cohort," *Nutrition Journal* 13 (99) (2014). https://www.ncbi.nlm.nih.gov/pmc/articles/PMC4209065/#__ffn_sectile, doi: 10.1186/1475 2891 13 99.

9   David Perlmutter, *Grain Brain* (New York: Little, Brown and Company, 2013), 32.

10   A. Rubio Tapia, J.F. Ludvigsson, T.L. Brantner, J.A. Murray, J.E. Everhart, "The Prevalence of Celiac Disease in the United States," *American Journal of Gastroenterology*, 107 (10) (2012):1538 44 doi: 10.1038/ajg.2012.219.

11   D.V. DiGiacomo, C.A. Tennyson, P.H. Green, R.T. Demmer, "Prevalence of Gluten Free Diet Adherence Among Individuals Without Celiac Disease in the USA: Results from the Continuous National Health and Nutrition Examination Survey 2009 2010", *Scandinavian Journal of Gastroenterology*, 48 (8) (2013): 921 5. doi: 10.3109/00365521.2013.809598.

12   The NPD Group, Inc., *Percentage of U.S. Adults Trying to Cut Down or Avoid Gluten in Their Diets Reaches New High in 2013, Reports NPD* (press release), https://www.npd.com/wps/portal/npd/us/news/press releases/percentage of US adults trying to cut down or avoid gluten in their diets reaches new high in 2013 reports npd/.

13   A. Capannolo et al., "Non Celiac Gluten Sensitivity among Patients Perceiving Gluten Related Symptoms," *Digestion* 92 (1) (2015): 8–13.

14   E. Q. Ye et al., "Greater Whole Grain Intake Is Associated with Lower Risk of Type 2 Diabetes, Cardiovascular Disease, and Weight Gain," *Journal of Nutrition* 142 (7) (2012): 1304–1313, doi: 10.3945/jn.111.155325.

15   D. Aune et al., "Whole Grain Consumption and Risk of Cardiovascular Disease, Cancer, and All Cause and Cause Specific Mortality: Systematic Review and Dose Response Meta Analysis of Prospective Studies" *BMJ* 353 (i2716) (2016). doi: 10.1136/bmj.i2716.

16   Geng Zong, Alisa Gao, Frank B. Hu, and Qi Sun, "Whole Grain Intake and Mortality from All Causes, Cardiovascular Disease, and Cancer," *Circulation* 133 (24) (2016): 2370–2380.

17   P. Tighe et al., "Effect of Increased Consumption of Whole Grain Foods on Blood Pressure and Other Cardiovascular Risk Markers in Healthy Middle Aged Persons: A Randomized Controlled Trial," *American Journal of Clinical Nutrition* 92 (4) (2010): 733–40, doi: 10.3945/ajcn.2010.29417.

18   A. D. Liese et al., "Whole Grain Intake and Insulin Sensitivity: The Insulin Resistance Atherosclerosis Study," *American Journal of Clinical Nutrition* 78 (5) (2003): 965–971.

19   Nicola M. McKeown et al., "Whole and Refined Grain Intakes Are Differentially Associated with Abdominal Visceral and Subcutaneous Adiposity in Healthy Adults: the Framingham Heart Study," *American Journal of Clinical Nutrition* 92 (5) (2010): 1165–1171.

20   Michael Lefevre and Satya Jonnalagadda, "Effect of Whole Grains on Markers of Subclinical Inflammation," *Nutrition Reviews* 70 (7) (2012): 387–396, doi: 10.1111/j.1753 4887.2012.00487.x.

21   Robert A. Vogel et al., "Effect of a Single High Fat Meal on Endothelial Function in Healthy Subjects," *American Journal of Cardiology* 79 (3) (1997): 350–354; Jukka Montonen et al., "Consumption of Red Meat and Whole Grain Bread in Relation to Biomarkers of Obesity, Inflammation, Glucose Metabolism and Oxidative Stress," *European Journal of Nutrition* 52 (1) (2013): 337–345.

22   Michael Greger, in conversation with the authors, February 2016.

Chapter 8. The Caveman Cometh: Promises and Pitfalls of the Paleo Diet

1   Loren Cordain, *The Paleo Diet* (New York: John Wiley & Sons, 2010), 10.

2   Loren Cordain, 2014, "Dairy: Milking It for All It's Worth," accessed October 2016, http://thepaleodiet .com/dairy milking worth.

3   Hongyu Wu, PhD et al., "Association between Dietary Whole Grain Intake and Risk of Mortality: Two Large Prospective Studies in US Men and Women," *JAMA Internal Medicine* 175 (3) (2015): 373–384, doi:10.1001/jamainternmed.2014.6283.

4   I. Darmadi Blackberry et al., "Legumes: The Most Important Dietary Predictor of Survival in Older People of Different Ethnicities," *Asia Pacific Journal of Clinical Nutrition* 3 (2) (2004): 217–220.

5   World Cancer Research Fund International/American Institute for Cancer Research, "Food, Nutrition, Physical Activity, and the Prevention of Cancer: A Global Perspective," Washington, D.C.: AICR, 2007.

6   Marlene Zuk, *Paleofantasy: What Evolution Really Tells Us about Sex, Diet, and How We Live* (New York: WW Norton & Company, 2013), 120.

7   Christina Warriner, "Debunking the Paleo Diet," Talk at TedX OU, http://tedxtalks.ted.com/video/ Debunking the Paleo Diet Christ.

8   Nathaniel J. Dominy, in conversation with John McDougall, MD, McDougall Advanced Study Weekend, Sept. 10, 2011, https://www.youtube.com/watch?v=ufNEoLeVplc.

9   Ann Gibbons, "Evolution of Diet," National Geographic, accessed October 2016, http://www .nationalgeographic.com/foodfeatures/evolution of diet.

10   Amanda G. Henry, Alison S. Brooks, and Dolores R. Piperno, "Microfossils in Calculus Demonstrate Consumption of Plants and Cooked Foods in Neanderthal Diets (Shanidar III, Iraq; Spy I and II, Belgium)" *Proceedings of the National Academy of Sciences* 108 (2) (2011): 486–491, doi:10.1073/ pnas.1016868108.

11   Melvin Konner, "Confessions of a Paleo Pioneer," *Wall Street Journal*, January 20, 2016, http://www.wsj .com/articles/an evolutionary guide revised on what to eat 1453306447.

12   Ibid.

13   David Katz, "Humanity's Fishy Origins," *Huffington Post*, September 8, 2016, http://www.huffingtonpost .com/entry/humanitys fishy origins or the paleo elephant in_us_57d1b639e4b0f831f7071735.

14   Susanna C. Larsson and Nicola Orsini, "Red Meat and Processed Meat Consumption and All Cause Mortality: A Meta Analysis," *American Journal of Epidemiology* 179 (3) (2014): 282–289, doi:10.1093/aje/ kwt261.

PART II. THE WHOLE FOODIE LIFESTYLE

Chapter 9. So, What Should I Eat? Navigating Everyday Food Choices

1   Trisha Ward, 2016, "Dean Ornish in Defense of the Dietary Fat Heart Disease Link," Medscape, May 12, 2016, accessed September 2016, http://www.medscape.com/viewarticle/862903.

2   Pam Popper, in conversation with the authors, May 2016.

3   Davis, *Proteinaholic*, 273.

4   Michael Pollan, *In Defense of Food: An Eater's Manifesto* (New York, NY: Penguin, 2009) 156–157.

5   2015, "Q&A on the Carcinogenicity of the Consumption of Red Meat and Processed Meat," World Health Organization, accessed September 2016, http://www.who.int/features/qa/cancer red meat/en/.

6   M. Song et al., "Association of Animal and Plant Protein Intake with All Cause and Cause Specific Mortality," *JAMA Internal Medicine* 176 (10) (2016): 1453–1463, doi:10.1001/jamainternmed.2016.4182.

7   Jennifer J. Otten, Jennifer Pitzi Hellwig, and Linda D. Meyers, eds., *National Academy Dietary reference intakes: the essential guide to nutrient requirements,* (Washington DC: The National Academies Press, 2006) 144.

8   U.S. Department of Agriculture, Agricultural Research Service. 2008. Nutrient Intakes from Food: Mean Amounts and Percentages of and Alcohol, One Day, 2005 2006. Available: https://www.ars.usda.gov/

ARSUserFiles/80400530/pdf/1314/Table_1_NIN_GEN_13.pdf.

9 Davis, *Proteinaholic*, 74.

10 Ibid., 7.

11 W. J. Craig, A. R. Mangels, "Position of the American Dietetic Association: Vegetarian Diets," *Journal of the American Dietetic Association* 109 (7) (2009): 1266–1282.

12 A. P. Simopoulos, "The Importance of the Ratio of Omega 6/Omega 3 Essential Fatty Acids," *Biomedicine & Pharmacotherapy* 56 (8) (2002): 365–379.

13 R. Pamplona and G. Barja, "An Evolutionary Comparative Scan for Longevity Related Oxidative Stress Resistance Mechanisms in Homeotherms," *Biogerontology* 12 (2011): 409 435, doi:10.1007/s10522 011 9348 1.

14 C. V. Felton et al., "Dietary Polyunsaturated Fatty Acids and Composition of Human Aortic Plaques," *Lancet* 344 (8931) (1994): 1195–1196, doi: http://dx.doi.org/10.1016/S0140 6736(94)90511 8; D. H. Blankenhorn et al., "The Influence of Diet on the Appearance of New Lesions in Human Coronary Arteries," *Journal of the American Medical Association* 263 (12) (1990): 1646–1652.

15 J. Connor, "Alcohol Consumption as a Cause of Cancer," *Addiction* (2016): doi: 10.1111/add.13477. http://onlinelibrary.wiley.com/doi/10.1111/add.13477/abstract.

16 R. Reiss, J. Johnston, K. Tucker, J.M. DeSesso, C.L. Keen, "Estimation of Cancer Risks and Benefits Associated with a Potential Increased Consumption of Fruits And Vegetables, Food and Chemical Toxicology 50 (12) (2012) 4421 7. doi: 10.1016/j.fct.2012.08.055.

17 Weaver CM, Plawecki KL, "Dietary calcium: adequacy of a vegetarian diet," Am J Clin Nutr. 1994 May;59(5 Suppl):1238S 1241S.

18 E. Madry, A. Lisowska, P. Grebowiec, J. Walkowiak, "The Impact of Vegan Diet on B 12 Status in Healthy Omnivores: Five Year Prospective Study," *Acta Scientiarum Polonorum Technologia Alimentaria* 11 (2) (2012): 209–212; M. S. Donaldson, "Metabolic Vitamin B12 Status on a Mostly Raw Vegan Diet with Follow Up Using Tablets, Nutritional Yeast, or Probiotic Supplements," *Annals of Nutrition and Metabolism*, 44 (5–6) (2000): 229–234; I. Elmadfa, and I. Singer, "Vitamin B 12 and Homocysteine Status among Vegetarians: A Global Perspective," *American Journal of Clinical Nutrition*, 89 (5) (2009): 1693S–1698S, doi: 10.3945/ajcn.2009.26736Y; A. M. Gilsing et al., "Serum Concentrations of Vitamin B12 and Folate in British Male Omnivores, Vegetarians and Vegans: Results from a Cross Sectional Analysis of the EPIC Oxford Cohort Study," *European Journal of Clinical Nutrition* 64 (9) (2010): 933–939, doi: 10.1038/ejcn.2010.142.

19 Roman Pawlak et al., "Understanding Vitamin B12," *American Journal of Lifestyle Medicine*, published online June 20, 2012, doi: 10.1177/1559827612450688; C. Chalouhi et al., "Neurological Consequences of Vitamin B12 Deficiency and Its Treatment," *Pediatric Emergency Care* 24 (8) (2008): 538–541, doi: 10.1097/PEC.0b013e318180ff32.; T. Kwok et al., "Vitamin B 12 Supplementation Improves Arterial Function in Vegetarians with Subnormal Vitamin B 12 Status," *Journal of Nutrition, Health and Aging* 16 (6) (2012): 569–573; D. K. Dror and L. H. Allen, "Effect of Vitamin B12 Deficiency on Neurodevelopment in Infants: Current Knowledge and Possible Mechanisms," *Nutrition Reviews* 66 (5) (2008): 250–255, doi: 10.1111/j.1753 4887.2008.00031.x.

20 I. Volkov et al., "Modern Society and Prospects of Low Vitamin B12 Intake," *Annals of Nutrition and Metabolism* 51 (5) (2007): 468–470; L. H. Allen, "How Common is Vitamin B 12 Deficiency?" *American Journal of Clinical Nutrition* 89 (2) (2009): 693S–696S, doi: 10.3945/ajcn.2008.26947A; M. van Dusseldorp et al., "Risk of Persistent Cobalamin Deficiency in Adolescents Fed a Macrobiotic Diet in Early Life," *American Journal of Clinical Nutrition* 69 (4) (1999): 664–671.

21 Joanne L. Slavin and Beate Lloyd, "Health Benefits of Fruits and Vegetables," *Advances in Nutrition* 3 (4) (2012): 506–516, doi: 10.3945/an.112.002154.

22 J. R. Hunt, "Bioavailability of Iron, Zinc, and Other Trace Minerals from Vegetarian Diets," *American Journal of Clinical Nutrition* 78 (3 Suppl) (2003): 633S–639S; P. J. Tuso, M. H. Ismail, B. P. Ha, and C. Bartolotto, "Nutritional Update for Physicians: Plant Based Diets," *Permanente Journal* 17 (2) (2013): 61–66, doi: 10.7812/TPP/12 085; Kate Marsh, Carol Zeuschner, and Angela Saunders, "Health Implications of a Vegetarian Diet: A Review," *American Journal of Lifestyle Medicine* 6 (250) (2012): 250 267, doi: 10.1177/1559827611425762.

23 D. R. Jacobs Jr., J. Ruzzin, D. H. Lee, "Environmental Pollutants: Downgrading the Fish Food Stock Affects Chronic Disease Risk," *Journal of Internal Medicine* 276 (3) (2014): 240–242, doi: 10.1111/joim.12205; J. Ruzzin, D. R. Jacobs, "The Secret Story of Fish: Decreasing Nutritional Value Due to Pollution?" *British Journal of Nutrition* 108 (3) (2012): 397–399, doi: 10.1017/S0007114512002048; W. J. Crinnion, "Polychlorinated Biphenyls: Persistent Pollutants with Immunological, Neurological, and Endocrinological Consequences," *Alternative Medicine Review* 16 (1) (2011): 5–13.

24 D. F. Rawn et al., "Persistent Organic Pollutants in Fish Oil Supplements on the Canadian Market: Polychlorinated Biphenyls and Organochlorine Insecticides," *Journal of Food Science* 74 (1) (2009): T14–T19, doi: 10.1111/j.1750 3841.2008.01020.x; E. Hoh et al., "Simultaneous Quantitation of Multiple

Classes of Organohalogen Compounds in Fish Oils with Direct Sample Introduction Comprehensive Two Dimensional Gas Chromatography and Time of Flight Mass Spectrometry," *Journal of Agricultural and Food Chemistry* 57 (7) (2009): 2653–2660, doi: 10.1021/jf900462p.

25   A. A. Welch et al., "Dietary Intake and Status of n 3 Polyunsaturated Fatty Acids in a Population of Fish Eating and Non Fish Eating Meat Eaters, Vegetarians, and Vegans and the Product Precursor Ratio [Corrected] of Linolenic Acid to Long Chain n-3 Polyunsaturated Fatty Acids: Results from the EPIC Norfolk Cohort," *American Journal of Clinical Nutrition* 92 (5) (2010): 1040–1051, doi: 10.3945/ajcn.2010.29457.

26   A. V. Witte et al., "Long Chain Omega 3 Fatty Acids Improve Brain Function and Structure in Older Adults," *Cerebral Cortex* 24 (11) (2014): 3059–3068, doi: 10.1093/cercor/bht163; *Fats and fatty acids in human nutrition. Report of an expert consultation,* (Rome: Food and Agriculture Organization of the United States, 2010) 1 166.

27   B. Sarter, K. S. Kelsey, T. A. Schwartz, and W. S. Harris, "Blood Docosahexaenoic Acid and Eicosapentaenoic Acid in Vegans: Associations with Age and Gender and Effects of an Algal Derived Omega 3 Fatty Acid Supplement," *Clinical Nutrition* 34 (2) (2015): 212–218, doi: 10.1016/j.clnu.2014.03.003.

28   Ibid.

29   K. Lane, E. Derbyshire, W. Li, and C. Brennan, "Bioavailability and Potential Uses of Vegetarian Sources of Omega 3 Fatty Acids: A Review of the Literature," *Critical Reviews in Food Science and Nutrition* 54 (5) (2014): 572–579, doi: 10.1080/10408398.2011.596292.

30   M. Narce, J. P. Poisson, J. Bellenger, and S. Bellenger, "Effect of Ethanol on Polyunsaturated Fatty Acid Biosynthesis in Hepatocytes from Spontaneously Hypertensive Rats," *Alcoholism: Clinical and Experimental Research* 25 (8) (2001): 1231–1237; D. F. Horrobin, "A Biochemical Basis for Alcoholism and Alcohol Induced Damage Including the Fetal Alcohol Syndrome and Cirrhosis: Interference with Essential Fatty Acid and Prostaglandin Metabolism," *Medical Hypotheses* 6 (9) (1980): 929–942.

31   B. Lands, "Dietary Omega 3 and Omega 6 Fatty Acids Compete in Producing Tissue Compositions and Tissue Responses," *Military Medicine* 179 (11 Suppl) (2014): 76–81, doi: 10.7205/MILMED D 14 00149.

32   James V. Pottala et al. "Higher RBC EPA + DHA Corresponds with Larger Total Brain and Hippocampal Volumes: WHIMS MRI Study," *Neurology* 82 (5) (2014): 435–442.

33   A. Veronica Witte et al., "Long Chain Omega 3 Fatty Acids Improve Brain Function and Structure in Older Adults," *Cerebral Cortex* 24 (11) (2014): 3059–3068, doi:10.1093/cercor/bht163.

Chapter 10. The Essential Eight: Health-Promoting Foods to Eat Every Day

1   Monica H. Carlsen et al., "The Total Antioxidant Content of More than 3100 Foods, Spices, Beverages, Herbs and Supplements Used Worldwide," *Nutrition Journal* 9 (3) (2010).

2   George H. Perry, Nathaniel J. Dominy, Katrina G. Claw et al., "Diet and the Evolution of Human Amylase Gene Copy Number Variation," *Nature Genetics* 39 (10) (2007): 1256–1260.

3   Aune Dagfinn et al., "Whole Grain Consumption and Risk of Cardiovascular Disease, Cancer, and All Cause and Cause Specific Mortality: Systematic Review and Dose Response Meta Analysis of Prospective Studies," *BMJ* 353 (i2716) (2016).

4   Y. Papanikolaou and V. L. Fulgoni III, "Bean Consumption Is Associated with Greater Nutrient Intake, Reduced Systolic Blood Pressure, Lower Body Weight, and a Smaller Waist Circumference in Adults: Results from the National Health and Nutrition Examination Survey 1999–2002," *Journal of the American College of Nutrition* 27 (5) (2008): 569–576.

5   Vanessa Ha et al., "Effect of Dietary Pulse Intake on Established Therapeutic Lipid Targets for Cardiovascular Risk Reduction: A Systematic Review and Meta Analysis of Randomized Controlled Trials," *Canadian Medical Association Journal* (2014), doi: 10.1503/cmaj.131727. 186 (8), 252–262.

6   Dan Buettner, in conversation with the authors, July 2016.

7   I. Darmadi Blackberry et al., "Legumes: The Most Important Dietary Predictor of Survival in Older People of Different Ethnicities," *Asia Pacific Journal of Clinical Nutrition* 3 (2) (2004): 217–220.

8   A. H. Wu, M. C. Yu, C. C. Tseng, and M. C. Pike, "Epidemiology of Soy Exposures and Breast Cancer Risk," *British Journal of Cancer* 98 (1) (2008): 9–14; X. O. Shu et al., "Soy food intake and breast cancer survival," *Journal of the American Medical Association* 302 (22) (2009): 2437–2443.

9   L. Yan, E.L. Spitznagel, "Soy Consumption and Prostate Cancer Risk in Men: A Revisit of a Meta-Analysis, *American Journal of Clinical Nutrition,* 8 9(4) (2009) 1155-63.

10   Neal Barnard, MD, "Settling the Soy Controversy," *Huffington Post,* April 26, 2010, http://www.huffingtonpost.com/neal barnard md/settling the soy controve_b_453966.html.

11   Hong Mei Zhang et al., "Research Progress on the Anticarcinogenic Actions and Mechanisms of Ellagic Acid." *Cancer Biology & Medicine* 11 (2) (2014): 92–100.

12   E. E. Devore, J. H. Kang, M. M. B. Breteler, and F. Grodstein, "Dietary Intakes of Berries and Flavonoids in Relation to Cognitive Decline," *Annals of Neurology* 72 (1) (2012): 135–143, doi: 10.1002/ana.23594.

13   Iris Erlund et al., "Favorable Effects of Berry Consumption on Platelet Function, Blood Pressure, and

HDL Cholesterol," *American Journal of Clinical Nutrition* 87 (2) (2008): 323–331; M. L. McCullough et al., "Flavonoid Intake and Cardiovascular Disease Mortality in a Prospective Cohort of US Adults," *American Journal of Clinical Nutrition* 95 (2) (2012): 454–464.

14 Monica H. Carlsen et al., "The Total Antioxidant Content of More than 3100 Foods, Beverages, Spices, Herbs and Supplements Used Worldwide," *Nutrition Journal* 9 (3) (2010).

15 Isao Muraki et al., "Fruit Consumption and Risk of Type 2 Diabetes: Results from Three Prospective Longitudinal Cohort Studies," *BMJ* 347 (f5001) (2013).

16 Fuhrman, *Super Immunity*, 69.

17 G. Murillo and R. G. Mehta, "Cruciferous Vegetables and Cancer Prevention," *Nutrition and Cancer* 41 (1–2) (2001): 17–28.

18 H. C. Hung et al., "Fruit and Vegetable Intake and Risk of Major Chronic Disease," *Journal of the National Cancer Institute* 96 (21) (2004): 1577–1584.

19 P. Carter et al., "Fruit and Vegetable Intake and Incidence of Type 2 Diabetes Mellitus: Systematic Review and Meta Analysis," *BMJ* 341 (c4229) (2010).

20 Latetia Moore, Jordana Turkel, and Joy Dubost, "Adults Meeting Fruit and Vegetable Intake Recommendations—United States, 2013," *Morbidity and Mortality Weekly Report* 64 (26) (2015): 709–713.

21 Union of Concerned Scientists, *Extra Daily Serving of Fruits or Vegetables Can Save Lives and Billions in Health Care Costs* (press release), August 7, 2013, http://www.ucsusa.org/news/press_release/produce saves lives money 0398.html#.V2wgrFeHClw.

22 Joel Fuhrman, MD, 2016, "The Healthiest, Anti Cancer Foods: G BOMBS," accessed October 2016, https://www.drfuhrman.com/learn/library/articles/29/the healthiest anti cancer foods g bombs.

23 Emilio Ros, "Health Benefits of Nut Consumption," *Nutrients* 2 (7) (2010): 652–682; Ying Bao, MD, ScD et al., "Association of Nut Consumption with Total and Cause Specific Mortality," *New England Journal of Medicine* 369 (21) (2013): 2001–2011, doi: 10.1056/NEJMoa1307352; Emilio Ros and Frank B. Hu, "Consumption of Plant Seeds and Cardiovascular Health," *Circulation* 128 (5) (2013): 553–565, originally published July 29, 2013, http://dx.doi.org/10.1161/CIRCULATIONAHA.112.001119.

24 "The Adventist Health Study: Findings for Nuts," Loma Linda University, accessed October 2016, http://publichealth.llu.edu/adventist health studies/findings/findings past studies/adventist health study findings nuts.

25 J. Sabaté, "Nut Consumption and Body Weight," *American Journal of Clinical Nutrition* 78 (3 Suppl) (2003): 647S–650S.

Chapter 11. Healthier *and* Happier: The Psychology and Physiology of Food and Pleasure

1 Douglas J. Lisle, PhD and Alan Goldhamer, DC, *The Pleasure Trap: Mastering the Hidden Force That Undermines Health and Happiness* (Summertown, TN: Healthy Living Publications, 2006), 15.

2 Ibid., 21.

3 V. Bassareo and G. Di Chiara, "Differential Responsiveness of Dopamine Transmission to Food Stimuli in Nucleus Accumbens Shell/Core Compartments," *Neuroscience* 89 (3) (1999): 637–641.

4 A. Drewnowski, D.D. Krahn, M.A. Demitrack, K. Nairn, B.A. Gosnell, "Taste Responses and Preferences for Sweet High-Fat Foods: Evidence for Opioid Involvement," *Physiological Behavior*, 51 (2) (1992) 371-9.

5 E. Hazum, J.J. Sabatka, K.J. Chang, D.A. Brent, J.W. Findlay, P. Cuatrecasas, "Morphine in Cow and Human Milk: Could Dietary Morphine Constitute a Ligand for Specific Morphine (Mu) Receptors?" *Science*. 213 (4511) (1981) 1010-12; H. Meisel, R.J. FitzGerald, "Opioid Peptides Encrypted in Intact Milk Protein Sequences," *British Journal of Nutrition*, 84 (Suppl 1) (2000) 27-31.

6 Lisle and Goldhamer, *Pleasure Trap*, 89.

7 Ciara Rooney, Michelle C. McKinley, and Jayne V. Woodside, "The Potential Role of Fruit and Vegetables in Aspects of Psychological Well-Being: A Review of the Literature and Future Directions," *Proceedings of the Nutrition Society* 72 (4) (2013): 420 432, doi:10.1017/S0029665113003388.

8 B. A. White, C. C. Horwath, and T. S. Conner, "Many Apples a Day Keep the Blues Away—Daily Experiences of Negative and Positive Affect and Food Consumption in Young Adults," *British Journal of Health Psychology* 18 (4) (2013): 782–798, doi:10.1111/bjhp.12021.

9 T. S. Conner, K. L. Brookie, A. C. Richardson, and M. A. Polak, "On Carrots and Curiosity: Eating Fruit and Vegetables Is Associated with Greater Flourishing in Daily Life," *British Journal of Health Psychology* 20 (2) (2015): 413–427, doi:10.1111/bjhp.12113.

10 Michael Greger, 2016, "Which Foods Increase Happiness?" NutritionFacts.org, accessed October 2016, http://nutritionfacts.org/video/foods increase happiness.

11 B. A. White, C. C. Horwath, and T. S. Conner, "Many Apples a Day Keep the Blues Away—Daily Experiences of Negative and Positive Affect and Food Consumption in Young Adults," *British Journal of Health Psychology* 18 (4) (2013): 782–798, doi:10.1111/bjhp.12021.

Chapter 12. Making the Shift: Proven Strategies for Successful Transitions

1   Thomas Campbell, MD, *The China Study Solution: The Simple Way to Lose Weight and Reverse Illness, Using a Whole Food, Plant Based Diet* (New York: Rodale Books, 2016), 140.
2   Kathy Freston, *The Book of Veganish* (New York: Pam Krauss/Avery, 2016), 113.
3   J. Holt Lunstad, T. B. Smith, J. B. Layton, "Social Relationships and Mortality Risk: A Meta Analytic Review," *PLOS Medicine* 7 (7): e1000316. doi: 10.1371/journal.pmed.1000316.
4   Pam Popper, in conversation with the authors, May 2016.
5   Matthew Lederman, MD, and Alona Pulde, MD, *The Forks over Knives Family: Every Parent's Guide to Raising Healthy, Happy Kids on a Whole Food, Plant Based Diet* (New York: Touchstone, 2016), 45.
6   Ibid., 48.
7   Ibid., 50.
8   Ibid., 51.
9   Ibid.
10   Pam Popper, in conversation with the authors, May 2016.

Chapter 13. Change Your Plate, Change the World

1   "Farm Animal Statistics: Slaughter Totals," the Humane Society of the United States, accessed October 2016, http://www.humanesociety.org/news/resources/research/stats_slaughter_totals. html?referrer=https://www.google.com.
2   Sir Paul McCartney, narrating PETA video *Glass Walls*, http://www.peta.org/videos/glass walls 2/.
3   Wayne Pacelle, *The Humane Economy: How Innovators and Enlightened Consumers Are Transforming the Lives of Animals* (New York: William Morrow, 2016), 280.
4   Colin Spencer, *Vegetarianism: A History* (New York: Four Walls Eight Windows, 2002), 43.
5   Jeremy Bentham, *An Introduction to the Principles of Morals and Legislation* (Minneola, New York: Dover Publications, 2007), 311.
6   Peter Singer, *Animal Liberation* (New York: Harper Perennial, 2009), 163.
7   Laura Wellesley, Catherine Happer, and Antony Froggatt, *Changing Climate, Changing Diets: Pathways to Lower Meat Consumption* (Chatham House Report), November 2015, https://www.chathamhouse.org/ sites/files/chathamhouse/publications/research/CHHJ3820%20Diet%20and%20climate%20change%20 18.11.15_WEB_NEW.pdf.
8   The Facts, Cowspiracy.com, accessed October 2016, http://www.cowspiracy.com/facts.
9   David Tilman and Michael Clark, "Global Diets Link Environmental Sustainability and Human Health," *Nature* 515 (27) (2014): 518 22, doi: 10.1038/nature13959.
10   The Facts, Cowspiracy.com, accessed October 2016, http://www.cowspiracy.com/facts.
11   Peter Singer, ed., *In Defense of Animals* (New York: Basil Blackwell, 1985), 10.
12   Albert Schweitzer, "The Evolution of Ethics," *Atlantic Monthly*, November 1958, 69–73.

PART III. THE 28-DAY EAT REAL FOOD PLAN

Chapter 14. 28 Days to Transform Your Health

1   Lani Muelrath, *The Plant-Based Journey* (Dallas, TX: BenBella Books, 2015), 58.

INDEX

ABOUT THE AUTHORS

John Mackey, cofounder and CEO of Whole Foods Market, has grown the natural and organic grocer to a $16 billion Fortune 500 company with more than 470 stores and 90,000 team members in three countries. The company has been included on *Fortune* magazine's "100 Best Companies to Work For" list for 20 consecutive years and ranked first in the food and drug store industry as part of the magazine's "Most Admired Companies" list in 2016.

While devoting his career to helping shoppers satisfy their lifestyle needs with quality natural and organic foods, Mackey has also focused on building a more conscious way of doing business. He was the visionary for the Whole Planet Foundation to help end poverty in developing nations, the Local Producer Loan Program to help local food producers expand their businesses, the Global Animal Partnership rating scale for humane farm animal treatment, and the Health Starts Here initiative to promote health and wellness.

Mackey has been recognized as one of *Fortune*'s "World's 50 Greatest Leaders," Ernst & Young's "Entrepreneur of the Year Overall Winner for the United States," Institutional Investor's "Best CEO in America," Barron's "World's Best CEO," MarketWatch's "CEO of the Year," *Fortune*'s "Businessperson of the Year," and *Esquire*'s "Most Inspiring CEO."

A strong believer in free market principles, Mackey cofounded the Conscious Capitalism Movement (consciouscapitalism.org) and coauthored the *New York Times* and *Wall Street Journal* bestseller *Conscious Capitalism:*